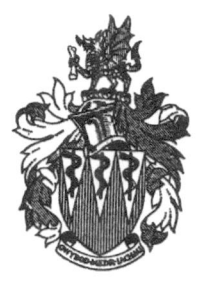

LYMPHORETICULAR MALIGNANCIES

LYMPHORETICULAR MALIGNANCIES

Epidemiologic and related aspects

N. J. VIANNA, MD, MSPH

Director, Lymphoma Research
Cancer Control Bureau
New York State Department of Health, Albany, New York

MTP
MEDICAL AND TECHNICAL
PUBLISHING CO LTD

Published by
MTP
MEDICAL AND TECHNICAL
PUBLISHING CO LTD
PO Box 55, St. Leonard's House
St. Leonard's Gate
Lancaster, Lancs.

ISBN 978-94-011-8055-9   ISBN 978-94-011-8053-5 (eBook)
DOI 10.1007/978-94-011-8053-5

First published 1975

Contents

From the river flows many streams into the ocean . . .
it is difficult to detect the main current

Preface

No disease can exist by itself but rather each must be viewed as the result of some specific interaction between man and his environment. This fact is appreciated even by people in the most primitive of civilisations and prompts them to ask the basic question: 'Why did I develop this disease'? The astute clinician goes beyond establishing a diagnosis and asks similar questions of himself and his patient. Frequently a singular observation resulting from this type of inquiry provides the working hypothesis for the epidemiologist who again asks the same question, not of the individual but of a definable population at risk. As a science, epidemiology is bound to the laws of logic and statistics, but clearly it must go beyond this point. The epidemiologist faced with a statistically significant observation must also question its biologic relevance. He must evaluate the consistency of his findings with the more established features of the disease under study. He must also be sufficiently imaginative to challenge his results with additional studies, different in their methodologic approach; and, of great importance, he must have the courage to be wrong. But epidemiologic studies alone can never determine the specific aetiology of a disease. Other scientific disciplines with their own inherent limitations are also required. Thus, in cancer research, the laboratory investigator frequently employs animal models, but the applicability of results obtained to humans is always subject to question. This defines another challenge for the cancer epidemiologist in particular: to identify situations in the community that are capable of being studied in the laboratory.

Of the many different malignant diseases, this is an opportune time to study primary lymphoreticular disorders because various medical disciplines have recently contributed new information concerning the pathogenesis and aetiology of these diseases.

This book does not exhaustively review the subject matter of lymphoreticular malignancies, but rather it places major emphasis on recent developments in the epidemiology of this group of disorders. It also takes a broad view of recent contributions made by other scientific disciplines with the hope that the student of lymphoreticular malignancies might synthesise available information into a workable whole from which future hypotheses might be generated. The first chapter reviews the evidence suggesting that environmental factors might be important in various lymphoproliferative malignancies. Specific hypotheses have been advanced for certain disorders, such as Hodgkin's disease, Burkitt's lyphoma and acute lymphatic leukaemia of childhood, and accordingly individual chapters have been devoted to these subjects. A much broader approach must be taken with the other lymphoreticular disorders since our knowledge is less specific. In this circumstance, consideration has been given to several questions which I consider of central importance to our understanding of the other lymphomas: Is the present classification meaningful and if so what are its limitations? Are there major differences between these disorders and Hodgkin's disease which is grouped with them? Considering available information, is there any central theme which pertains to the other lymphomas? Another section of this book has been devoted to the childhood lymphomas. Although these diseases may be indistinguishable histologically in the young and old, a sufficient number of differences are present both between and within various age groups to warrant considering them separately.

The final chapter deals with factors which might predispose to certain lymphoreticular malignancies. It is hoped that this section will provide a basic framework for future studies. The great diversity in the types of factors identified, both real and potential, poses a clear challenge to the student of lymphomas, one that must not go unanswered.

ACKNOWLEDGEMENTS

I am indebted to the many patients I have met for their co-operation. I thank Doctors P. Greenwald and J. N. P. Davies for their encouragement and scientific advice and Judith Brady and Patricia Leveille for their technical assistance.

CHAPTER 1

Lymphoreticular malignancies as environmental disorders

Information of considerable importance has been gained from comparisons of the incidence of various malignant diseases, both between and within various populations. Although the role of hereditary factors can never be completely excluded, it is likely that the vast majority of the geographic differences observed for most cancers are environmentally induced. This would also appear to be true of the lymphomas and leukaemias, which are characterised by markedly diverse international patterns. When differences in incidence are polarised to the extent that a disease occurs only or mainly in relatively circumscribed areas, as is true with Burkitt's lymphoma, this allows one to concentrate on the differences between regions of high and low incidence. Do these areas differ mainly with respect to their physical environment (e.g. climate, geology), biologic environment or both? It must be realised, however, that it is difficult to dissect man from his environment; just as the nutritional, hygienic and socio-economic standards set by man can alter his environment so too existing physical and biologic factors can dramatically affect his activities. Despite all its uses, geographic epidemiology has its limitations, largely due to the lack of suitable statistics from certain areas, especially more primitive ones, and under ascertainment of cases which may be a function of the diagnostic facilities available. It is therefore imperative that other methods be employed in evaluating the possibility that a disease is environmentally induced. These include time–space cluster analysis, migration studies and evaluation of peculiar situations such as familial aggregations of a disease. Again each method has its own limitations so that a variety of approaches must be taken to adequately evaluate this question. This chapter examines the evidence that environmental factors might be important in the aetiology of certain lymphoreticular disorders.

HODGKIN'S DISEASE

Marked differences in the frequency of Hodgkin's disease have been observed both on the international level and regionally within certain countries (MacMahon, 1966). Variations have also been noted in overall rates and when such factors as age and sex are considered separately. In the United States (Figure 1.1) overall rates are higher than in Japan

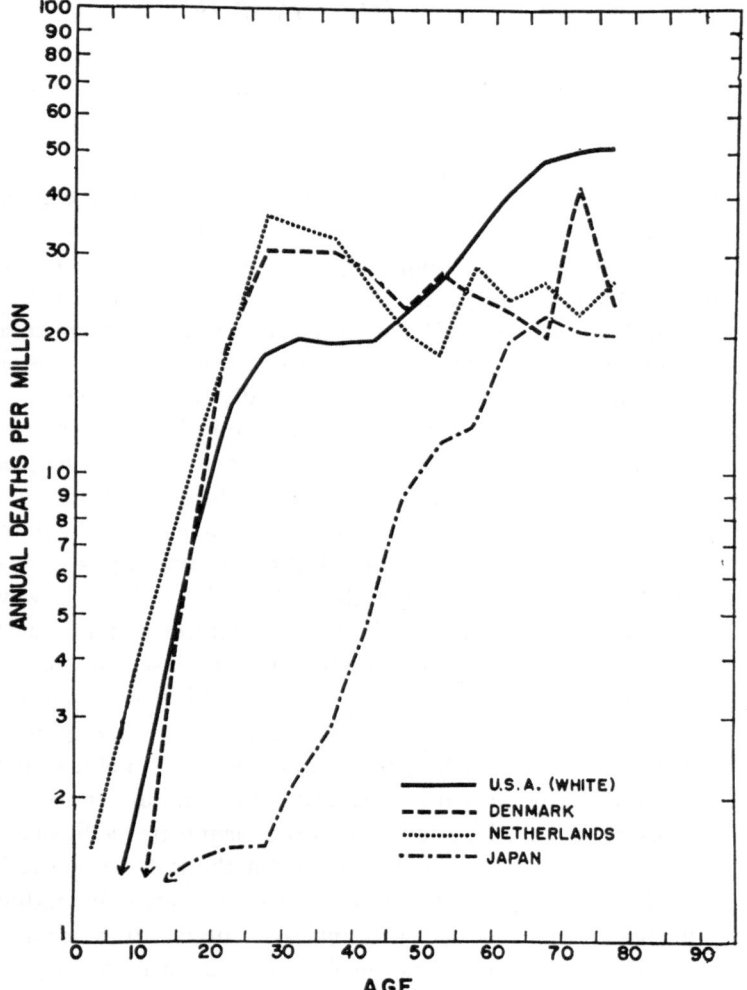

Figure 1.1 Age specific death rates from Hodgkin's disease in four countries, 1950–53. (From MacMahon, B. (1966), by courtesy of *Cancer Res.*)

and the age–specific incidence curve is characteristically bimodal. Similar bimodal curves have been observed in Great Britain (Stalsberg, 1972), Israel (Meytes and Modan, 1969), Denmark, the Netherlands (MacMahon, 1966), Northern Germany (Dörken and Singer-Bakker, 1972) and virtually every urbanised Western country where it has been sought. In Japan, the childhood age peak is clearly lacking whereas in Peru and Lebanon it predominates (Correa and O'Conor, 1971). Available data suggests that Hodgkin's disease accounts for a lower proportion of the lymphomas in Uganda than in the United States and Great Britain, but a higher proportion than found in Japan (Wright, 1973). These differences while dramatic, are difficult to intepret alone. But the evidence that Hodgkin's disease is primarily an environmentally induced malady goes beyond this point. Several studies have suggested that socio-economic factors play an important role with respect to the incidence of this disease. In the United States the disease appears to be associated with high socio-economic status among patients of 15 years of age and over (MacMahon, 1966). Unfortunately little is known about the importance of this factor for the younger age group in this country. This is a consideration of some importance since reports from other countries, especially in South America, suggest that the incidence of this disease is high among male children from poor areas (Correa and O'Conor, 1971). The importance of socio-economic factors is further suggested by the observation of three age incidence patterns for Hodgkin's disease, each apparently associated with different levels of economic development. The first pattern occurs primarily in developing countries as Peru and Columbia and is characterised by rates which are high among male children, low in the third decade of life and high in the older age groups. In urbanised countries rates are low in childhood but high for young adults and the elderly. An intermediate pattern, found in rural areas of developing countries such as Puerto Rico (Correa, 1972), is characterised by incidence rates which are somewhat higher in male children but lower in young adult males than those recorded in urbanised countries.

Leaving international comparisons for studies in specific regions, other important differences become apparent. Thus, MacMahon (1966) showed that between 1943 and 1957 the incidence of Hodgkin's disease among Danish males under 49 years of age, was higher in rural regions than in capital and suburban regions. Similar observations have been made by Dörken and Singer-Bakker (1972) in Northern Germany, and Fasal et al. (1968) noted that incidence rates are higher at younger ages among Californian male farm workers and Norwegian male rural residents. Still other studies have demonstrated significant variations in Hodgkin's disease mortality rates for different regions of the United States. Cole *et al.* (1968) studied eleven contiguous southern states from 1949–54 and 1959–61 and found mortality rates in young adults to be significantly lower than those recorded in the North. This 'Southern pattern' appeared to be characterised then by mortality rates approximating the national average for the older age groups but below it for the young adult age group. These intriguing observations raise a question of fundamental importance: what were the characteristics of the childhood mortality pattern in the South? This is partially answered by Fraumeni and Li (1969) who found higher childhood mortality rates in this region than in the North, albeit during a slightly different time period. The high childhood–low young adult–high older age group pattern suggested by these studies corresponds best to that observed for developing countries. Are the different age distributions observed in various small countries primarily a reflection of the multiplicity of patterns occurring in different regions of a large country? Unfortunately this crucial question has not been satisfactorily answered at present. The obvious implication of the international, regional, socio-economic and urban–rural differences observed however, is that all these factors are interrelated and might be explained by differing interactions between environment and host.

The results of various migration studies would also appear to be consistent with an environmental interpretation in Hodgkin's disease. In a recent study (Figure 1.2), age–specific mortality rates for Japanese-Americans were found to be higher than those for Japan (Mason and Frauneri, 1974). This excess in mortality was statistically significant for the 15–34 and 50 and older age groups. Haenszel and Kurihara (1968) found standard mortality rates for Isei males and females to be more closely aligned to those for United States' whites than for Japanese. Furthermore, there does not appear to be any significant difference in mortality rates between whites and Japanese living in Hawaii (Blaisdell and Boxer, 1971). Meytes and Modan (1969) found no significant difference in the incidence of Hodgkin's disease among various Israeli migrant populations, but they did observe that the bimodality was more pronounced for American, European and Asiatic born Jews than for those born in Africa.

The results of time-space cluster analysis in Hodgkin's disease have been quite variable. Thus reports by Gilmore and Telesnick (1962),

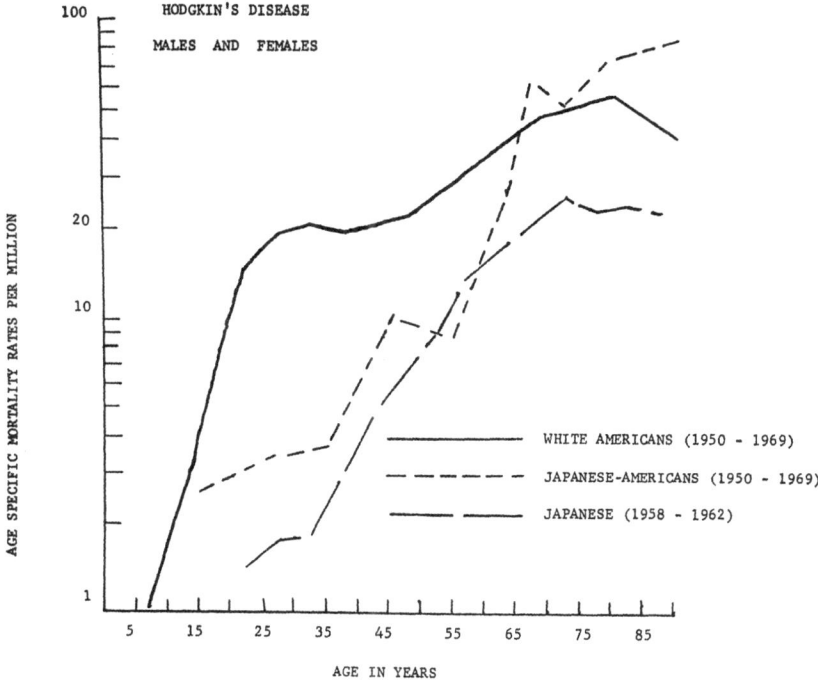

Figure 1.2 Mortality rates for Hodgkin's disease among US White and Japanese populations (1950–69) and native Japanese (1958–62) (From Mason, T. J. and Fraumeni, J. F. (1974) by courtesy of *Lancet*)

Clemmesen *et al.* (1952) and Bjelke (1969) would suggest that this phenomenon does occur whereas the more elaborate studies conducted by Alderson and Nayak (1971) found no overall evidence of clustering. Why should these discrepancies exist? While it is possible that clustering does not occur in Hodgkin's disease, the negative results obtained might be due in great part to the various time-space co-ordinates being rather arbitrarily chosen, the different age groups studied and the methods of analysis employed. Perhaps at this point it would be worth while to mention the obvious: all that encompasses the biologic world, including patients with Hodgkin's disease, is bound in time and space and each of these parameters represent a continuum of multiple points. If the reasonable assumption is made that Hodgkin's disease might have relatively specific aetiologic time and space co-ordinates, one is immediately confronted with two alternate approaches: either to continually select different co-ordinates at random from a pool of overwhelming combinations or to critically examine reported groupings of this disease for

probable co-ordinates, despite the fact that the biologic significance of
these groupings remains to be determined. The latter choice would
appear to be the more logical one, but has yet to be employed. More
will be said about the problems encountered in applying time-space
cluster analysis to Hodgkin's disease in Chapter 2.

Evaluation of familial aggregates of Hodgkin's disease provides
another means of crudely dissecting genetic disorders with a definite age
association from those primarily environmental in aetiology. Thus, if the
interval between diagnoses or onsets of illness is shorter than the age
(at diagnosis or onset) difference between two sibs, an environmental
interpretation is favoured (MacMahon, 1966). Although there have been
numerous reports of familial Hodgkin's disease, mostly sib–sib pairs
(MacMahon, 1966; Razis *et al.*, 1959; DeVore and Doan, 1957),
unfortunately the time interval between cases is not stated. While the
most detailed study of this type, that of Razis and his colleagues (1959),
presents evidence to favour environmental rather than genetic factors, it
has been pointed out that certain biases might account for these results.
In any hospital based study that employs a review of medical records to
detect familial cases, it is possible that cases occurring within a short
time interval would most likely be remembered and thus recorded in
preference to more distant ones. Furthermore, the statement of a patient
with Hodgkin's disease that he has a relative with the same disease is
unacceptable unless the diagnosis can be confirmed histologically. One
method of avoiding these confounding factors is to use tumour registries
or regional hospital surveys to identify familial cases with similar surnames, over long periods of time. This approach is limited by the fact
that it can not identify all familial cases, but it can be used as an objective means of determining the age and time intervals between such
cases. A recently conducted study of this type (Vianna *et al.*, 1974)
identified twenty-three familial pairs with Hodgkin's disease all of
which were reassessed histologically. Analysis of these pairs showed
that the time interval between diagnoses was shorter than the age
interval, thereby suggesting that environmental factors might be more
important than genetic. Taken together, the implication of these studies
and the international, regional and socio-economic differences observed
seems clear; environmental factors undoubtedly play a major role in the
aetiology of Hodgkin's disease.

OTHER LYMPHORETICULAR DISORDERS

In contrast to Hodgkin's disease, our knowledge of the epidemiology of the other lymphomas is quite limited. One major reason for this is the difficulty encountered in the classification of this group of disorders. For example, the histologic features of reticulum cell sarcoma are not pathognomonic and it is frequently difficult to distinguish this disorder from certain types of lymphosarcoma (Oéttlé, 1964). Furthermore, the validity of any histologic classification depends upon a certain constancy of morphology and cell types. Custer and Bernhard (1948) claimed that transitions from one type of lymphoma (including Hodgkin's disease) to other types occurs with some frequency. In contrast, Gall and Mallory (1942) and Rappaport (1966) were impressed with the general constancy of the various types of lymphoma. While the latter view is generally accepted, a more detailed classification which considers not only architecture and cell type but also recent immunologic concepts, will be required before this matter can be evaluated sufficiently. Despite these limitations, available evidence does suggest the importance of environmental factors in the non-Hodgkin's lymphomas. They apparently occur with a greater frequency and at earlier ages in Egypt than in America or European countries (El-Gazayerli *et al.*, 1962). In Uganda, there is a relatively high proportion of reticulum cell sarcoma (Table 1.1) and low proportion of lymphosarcoma and Hodgkin's disease when compared to the United States. The distribution of malignant lymphomas in Great Britain is similar to that observed in the United States (Wright, 1973), but the pattern in Japan (Anderson *et al.*, 1970) is more closely aligned with that of Uganda (Table 1.1). In Latin American countries, the

Table 1. 1. **Distribution of various lymphomas based on reports from different countries**

	Hodgkin's disease (%)	Lymphosarcoma (%)	Reticulum cell sarcoma (%)
United States			
Gall and Mallory (1942)	37·0	35·6	20·4
Jackson and Parker (1947)	32·6	43·3	19·6
Mollander and Pack (1963)	34·6	30·2	22·3
Japan			
Anderson *et al.* (1970)	16·2	14·3	64·4
Uganda			
Wright (1973)	18·5	19·2	23·7

frequency of Hodgkin's disease appears to be higher than that of reticulum cell sarcoma and lymphosarcoma (Besuschio, 1974). In Africa and New Guinea, the Burkitt lymphoma is very common (Krüger and O'Conor, 1972), in the United States and Great Britain it is quite rare and in tropical regions of Latin America, the incidence of this tumour is low to moderate (Besuschio, 1974). Interesting regional differences have also been observed for certain lymphomas. In Kyadondo County, Uganda, the overall incidence of lymphosarcoma is low when compared to Western countries, but rates for males with this disorder and Hodgkin's disease are higher in the Northern Province (Figure 1.3) than in Buganda, where medical facilities are better (Amsel and Nabembezi, 1974). These international and regional differences and the observation that the standard mortality ratios for Isei males and females are more similar to those for the white population in the United States (Haenszel and Kurihara, 1968), regardless of age, suggest that environmental factors are important in the group of disorders.

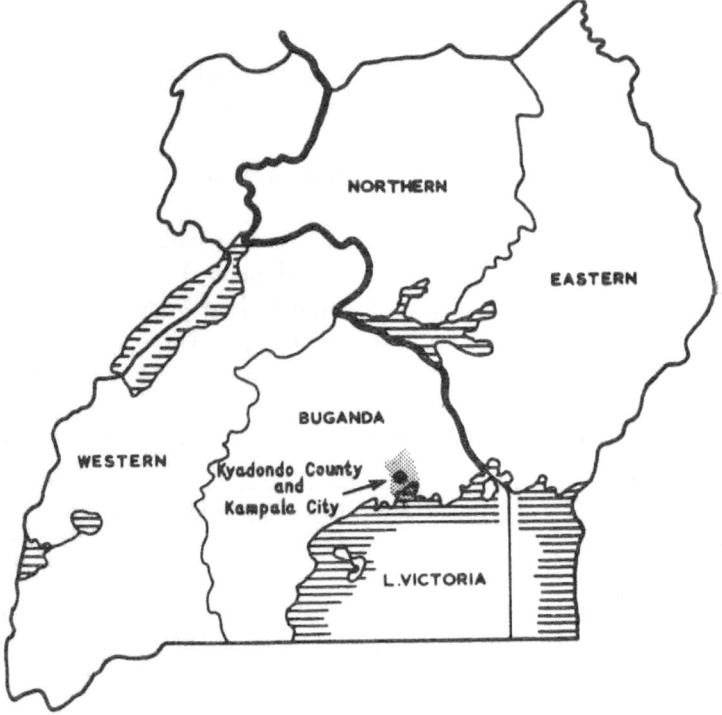

Figure 1.3 Map of Uganda showing the four provinces, Kyadondo County, and the capital, Kampala (from Amsel, S. and Nabembezi, J. S. (1974), by courtesy of *J. Nat. Cancer Inst.*)

International studies have also made us aware of specific features of the non-Hodgkin's lymphomas in certain areas. There is a close overlap of the Burkitt tumour belt with the classical malaria zones in Africa (Daldorf *et al.*, 1964; Burkitt, 1969). Is this mere coincidence or does the malaria parasite act as a chronic antigenic stimulus or immuno-suppressive agent which sets the stage for the Burkitt tumour (Krüger and O'Conor, 1972)? Lymphomas occur with great frequency among individuals under 20 years of age in Egypt. Is this possibly due to some relationship with chronic bilharziasis, which produces a marked reticulum cell proliferation in nodes draining active lesions (El-Gazayerli *et al.*, 1962)? There is a high frequency of intestinal lymphoma which appears to be related to high IgA levels in Arabs (Ramot and Many, 1972). Does chronic parasitic infection stimulate the gastrointestinal tract and ultimately lead to the development of intestinal lymphoma? In South America, splenic, follicular and nasal lymphomas appear to occur with undue frequency (Weiss and Morón, 1962; Andrade and Waldeck, 1971). Could this be due to customs specific to this area or environmental factors which tend to localise these disorders? These questions are worthy of further investigation. They all raise the possi-bility that specific environmental factors in certain areas might affect the incidence and/or mode of presentation of certain lymphoreticular disorders. The possibility must be considered that the same type of lymphoma may be associated with different factors in various parts of the world. For example, chronic parasitism may be a major predisposing factor to intestinal lymphomas in Arabian countries, but in Western countries, oeliac sprue might act in this capacity (Harris *et al.*, 1967).

In considering the lymphatic leukaemias, a major problem has been the fact that many previous studies did not treat each subtype separately. This is unfortunate since several studies (Court Brown and Doll, 1961; MacMahon and Clark, 1956; Fraumeni *et al.*, 1971) have suggested that each subtype has certain distinctive features. In general, leukaemia in Western countries has an age incidence peak before the fifth year of life, declines gradually during the middle years and then increases sharply with advanced age. In contrast, leukaemia in Uganda is not characterised by a childhood peak and rates decline after the age of 65 years (Amsel and Nabembezi, 1974). The absence of this early age peak is undoubtedly reflective of the low incidence of acute lymphatic leukaemia in this country (Amsel and Nabembezi, 1974; Templeton, 1973). In addition to the differences in leukaemia patterns that have been observed, other studies suggest the potential importance of environmental factors in the aetiology of acute lymphatic leukaemia. Knox (1964) suggested that seasonal factors might be more important in this subtype of childhood leukaemia than in the myeloid variety. Furthermore, it has been shown that the 3–4-year age peak, characteristically attributable to acute lymphatic leukaemia, occurred for the first time around 1920 in England (Court Brown and Doll, 1961) but around 1940 in the United States. In the United States the appearance of this peak depended as much on an increase in rates for the 3–4-year age group (Slocumb and MacMahon, 1963) as a decrease for those under 2 years of age. Furthermore, the first decline in overall leukaemia rates was observed during the period 1961–65 among United States whites but not among the non-white population (Fraumeni and Miller, 1967). Although this decline affected all ages between one and 75 years, it was most pronounced among children of 4 years or less. These rather dynamic changes represent important clues to childhood leukaemia; if for example the lymphatic subtype is attributable to environmental factors, these factors should vary concomitantly with changes in leukaemia trends. The important question, however, is whether the prenatal, natal or postnatal periods (or various combinations) represent the crucial time(s) of exposure. This concept will be discussed further in the chapter dealing with acute lymphatic leukaemia.

In contrast to acute lymphatic leukaemia, it is doubtful that chronic lymphatic leukaemia ever occurs in children. The incidence curve for this disorder increases rapidly with age and closely parallels the age incidence pattern of all lymphomas (MacMahon, 1966). It is extremely rare in Chinese and other Orientals (Wells and Lau, 1960) when compared with the rates in the United States and England. While the reasons for these international differences are unknown, it seems unlikely that they can be explained solely by genetic factors. Preliminary evidence suggests that the mortality due to this disorder among Chinese-Americans has not differed significantly from that observed for other Americans (Fraumeni and Mason, 1974).

References

Alderson, M. R. and Nayak, R.: A study of space-time clustering of Hodgkin's disease in the Manchester region. *Brit. J. Prev. Soc. Med.*, **25**:168, 1971.

Amsel, S. and Nabembezi, J. S.: Two-year survey of haematologic malignancies in Uganda. *J. Nat. Cancer Inst.*, **52**:1397, 1974.

Anderson, R. E., Ishida, K., Li, Y. *et al.*: Geographica spects of malignant lymphoma and multiple myeloma. *Amer. J. Pathol.*, **61**:85, 1970.

Andrade, Z. and Waldeck, N. A.: Follicular lymphoma of the spleen in patients with hepatosplenic Schistosomiasis mansoni. *Amer. J. Trop. Med. Hyg.*, 20:237, 1971.

Besuschio, S. C.: Geographic pathology of lymphomas in Latin America. *Medicina*, 34:31, 1974.

Bjelke, E.: Hodgkin's disease in Norway. *Acta Med. Scand.*, 185:73, 1969.

Blaisdell, R. K. and Boxer, G. J.: In: *Scientific Contributions, Second Meeting of the Asian–Pacific Division of the International Society of Haematology* (Melbourne, 1971).

Burkitt, D. P.: Etiology of Burkitt lymphoma, an alternative hypothesis to a vectoral virus. *J. Nat. Cancer Inst.*, 42: 19, 1969.

Clemmesen, J., Busk, T. and Nielsen, A.: The topographical distribution of leukemia and Hodgkin's disease in Denmark, 1942–46. *Acta Radiol. (Ther.) (Stock.)*, 37:223, 1952.

Cole, P., MacMahon, B. and Aisenberg, A.: Mortality from Hodgkin's disease in the United States. *Lancet*, 2:1371, 1968.

Correa, P.: *Hodgkin's disease in Latin America, International Symposium on Hodgkin's Disease*, 36 Washington, D.C.; (US.. Government Printing Office, 1972, 9) (National Cancer Institute Monograph).

Correa, P and O'Conor, G. T.: Epidemiologic patterns of Hodgkin's disease. *Int. J. Cancer*, 8:192, 1971.

Court Brown, W. M. and Doll, R.: Leukemia in childhood and young adult life: trends in mortality in relation to etiology. *Brit. Med. J.*, 1:981, 1961.

Custer, R. P. and Bernhard, W. G.: The interrelationships of Hodgkin's disease and other lymphatic tumors. *Amer. J. Med. Sci.*, 216:725, 1948.

Daldorf, G., Linsell, C. A., Barnhart, F. E. *et al.*: An epidemiologic approach to lymphomas of African children and Burkitt's sarcoma of the jaws. *Perspect. Biol. Med.*, 7:435, 1964.

DeVore, J. W. and Doan, C. A.: A study of the Hodgkin's syndrome XII. Hereditary and epidemiologic aspects. *Ann. Int. Med.*, 47:300, 1957.

Dörken, H. and Singer-Bakker, H.: Hodgkin's disease in childhood—an epidemiologic study in Northern Germany. In: *Current Problems in the Epidemiology of Cancer and Lymphomas*, 235, 1st. ed. (E. Grundmann, and H. Tullinius, editors) (Berlin, Heidelberg, New York: Springer–Verlag, 1972).

El–Gazayerli, M., Khalil, H., Abdel, A. *et al.*: Observations on some bilharzial reactions. *Alex. Med. J.*, 8:434, 1962.

Fasal, E., Jackson, E. W. and Klauber, M. R.: Leukemia and lymphoma mortality and farm residence. *Amer. J. Epidemiol* 87:267, 1968.

Fraumeni, J. F. and Li, F. P.: Hodgkin's disease in childhood; an epidemiologic study. *J. Nat. Cancer Inst.*, 42:681, 1969.

Fraumeni, J. F., Manning, M. D. and Mitus, W. J.: Acute childhood leukemia: epidemiologic study by cell type of 1,263 cases at Childrens Cancer Research Foundation in Boston, 1947–65. *J. Nat. Cancer Inst.*, 46:461, 1971.

Fraumeni, J. F. and Mason, T. J.: Cancer mortality among Chinese Americans. *J. Nat. Cancer Inst.* 52:659, 1974.

Fraumeni, J. F. and Miller, R. W.: Leukemia mortality: downturn in the United States. *Science*, 155:1126, 1967.

Gall, E. A. and Mallory, T. B.: Malignant lymphoma. Clinicopathologic survey of 613 cases. *Amer. J. Pathol.* 18:381, 1942.

Gilmore, H. R. and Telesnick, G.: Environmental Hodgkin's disease and leukemia. *Penn. Med. J.*, 65:1047, 1962.

Haenszel, W. and Kurihara, M.: Studies of Japanese migrants. I. Mortality from cancer and other diseases among Japanese in the United States. *J. Nat. Cancer Inst.*, **40**:43, 1968.

Harris, O. D., Cooke, W. T., Thompson, H. *et al.*: Malignancy in Adult Coeliac Disease and Idiopathic Steatorrhoea. *Amer. J. Med.*, **42**:899, 1967.

Jackson, H. Jr and Parker, F. Jr: *Hodgkin's Disease and Allied Disorders* (New York: Oxford Univ. Press, 1947).

Knox, G.: Epidemiology of childhood leukemia in Northumberland and Durham. *Brit. J. Prev. Soc. Med.*, **18**:17, 1964.

Krüger, G. and O'Conor, G. T.: Epidemiologic and Immunologic considerations on the pathogenesis of Burkitt's tumor. In: *Current Problems in the Epidemiology of Cancer and Lymphomas*, 213 (E. Grundmann and H. Tullinius, editors) (Berlin, Heidelberg, New York: Springer–Verlag 1972).

MacMahon, B.: Epidemiology of Hodgkin's disease. *Cancer Res.*, **26**:1189, 1966.

MacMahon, B. and Clark, D.: Incidence of common forms of human leukemia. *Blood*, **11**:871, 1956.

Mason, T. J. and Fraumeni, J. F.: Hodgkin's disease among Japanese Americans. *Lancet*, **1**:215, 1974.

Meytes, D. and Modan, B.: Selected aspects of Hodgkin's disease in a whole community. *Blood*, **34**:91, 1969.

Molander, D. W. and Pack, G. T.: Lymphosarcoma. Choice of treatment and end results in 567 patients. *Rev. Surg.*, **20**:3, 1963.

Oéttlé, A. G.: Primary malignant neoplasms of the lymphoreticular tissues (200–3, 205): a histopathologic series from White and Bantu races in the Transvaal, 1949–1953. *Symposium on Lymphoreticular Tumors in Africa, Paris, 1963*, 24 (F. C. Roulet, editor) (Basel-New York: Karger, 1964).

Ramot, B. and Many, A.: Primary intestinal lymphoma. In: *Current Problems in the Epidemiology of Cancer and Lymphomas*, 194 (E. Grundmann and H. Tullinius, editors) (Berlin, Heidelberg, New York: Springer–Verlag 1972).

Rappaport, H.: Tumors of the hematopoietic system. *Atlas of Tumor Pathology, Section III, Fascicle 8* (Washington, D.C.: Armed Forces Institute of Pathology, 1966).

Razis, D. V., Diamond, H. D. and Craver, L. F.: Familial Hodgkin's disease: its significance and implications. *Ann. Int. Med.*, **51**:933, 1959.

Slocumb, J. C. and MacMahon, B.: Changes in mortality rates from leukemia in the first five years of life. *N. Eng. J. Med.*, **268**:922, 1963.

Stalsberg, H.: Hodgkin's disease in Western Europe: A review–In: *International Symposium on Hodgkin's Disease*, 36 (Washington, D.C.: U.S. Government Printing Office, 1972, 31) (National Cancer Institute Monograph).

Templeton, A. C.: Leukemia. In: *Tumors in A Tropical Country*, 300 (A. C. Templeton, editor) (Berlin, Heidelberg, New York: Springer–Verlag 1973).

Vianna, N. J., Davies, J. N. P., Polan, A. and Wolfgang, P.: Hodgkin's disease: an environmental and genetic disorder. *Lancet*, **11**:854, 1974.

Weiss, P. and Morón, J.: Linfomas (reticulosarcomas) nasales. *Dermatol. Rev. Mex.*, **6**:34, 1962.

Wells, R. and Lau, K. S.: Incidence of leukemia in Singapore and rarity of chronic lymphatic leukemia in Chinese. *Brit. Med. J.*, **1**:759, 1960.

Wright, D. H.: Lymphoreticular malignancies. In: *Tumors in a Tropical Country*, 270 (A. C. Templeton, editor) (Berlin, Heidelberg, New York: Springer–Verlag, 1973).

CHAPTER 2

Hodgkin's disease; its heterogeneous nature and possible infectious aetiology

Two issues have dominated epidemiologic studies of Hodgkin's disease in recent years. One centres around the heterogeneous nature of this disorder, whereas the other issue deals with possible infectious aetiology in Hodgkin's disease and the various studies used to test this hypothesis. It seems clear that these concepts are intimately related for they both deal with the question of aetiology. If Hodgkin's disease is a single infectious disorder, the different characteristics observed for certain age groups must be explained. If the disease first described by Thomas Hodgkin in 1832 represents more than one entity, the question then becomes in which age groups is it infectious, neoplastic, etc.? The limitations of epidemiology as a scientific tool become immediately apparent when one ponders over the ways of answering these questions. For example, epidemiologic studies alone can never prove or disprove in absolute terms the hypotheses that Hodgkin's disease is infectious in origin. The epidemiologist can however, present evidence suggesting that different age groups should be evaluated separately by the other scientific disciplines or that Hodgkin's disease behaves as an infectious disorder under certain circumstances. In reviewing the history of this disease, the inescapable fact is that we have been asking the same basic questions since the turn of the century. We will undoubtedly go full circle again unless each scientific discipline listens to the footsteps of the other modes of inquiry. This chapter provides no definitive answers to the important aetiologic questions raised but rather it examines those studies which suggest that Hodgkin's disease has many heterogeneous features, especially when childhood and adult cases are compared. The available evidence suggesting that this disorder might be infectious in nature is also reviewed.

HETEROGENEITY WITHIN HODGKIN'S DISEASE

In contrast to reticulum cell sarcoma, lymphosarcoma and Burkitt's lymphoma, which have always been regarded as neoplastic disorders, there has been incessant controversy over the nature of Hodgkin's disease. Hodgkin considered it to be a hypertrophic lymphatic disorder, whereas others, such as Wilks (1865), Mallory (1914) and Warthin (1931), thought it was infectious. Although Sternberg (1898) and Reed (1902) both described the same classical giant cells that appear in Hodgkin's disease, even they had differing views as to its nature; Sternberg thought it was a variant of tuberculosis and Reed considered it to be an inflammatory disorder. In more recent years, it has been hypothesised that Hodgkin's disease is more than one entity, possibly an infectious or inflammatory disorder in the young and neoplastic in the elderly.

Histologic features

The Rye classification of Hodgkin's disease has gained wide acceptance and is indicative of the pleomorphic nature of this disorder. Admittedly there is a well-recognised transition from lymphocyte predominance through mixed cellularity to the lymphocyte depleted stage (Strum and Rappaport, 1971a) but each of these subtypes have certain distinctive features with regard to their cellular composition. For example, the diagnosis of the lymphocyte predominance and depleted stages depends not only on the number and maturity of the lymphocytes present, but also on the character and frequency of Reed–Sternberg cells. Lymphocyte predominant Hodgkin's disease tends to remain localised in the cervical nodes for long periods, is usually associated with a favourable prognosis and occurs mostly in young males (Berard *et al.*, 1971). In contrast, lymphocyte depletion is more widespread in its initial anatomic distribution, the prognosis is poor and it occurs with greater frequency in the elderly (Berard *et al.*, 1971; Thomas and Berard, 1973). A recent study (Neiman *et al.*, 1973) described a rapidly fatal syndrome associated with this subtype, characterised by fever, pancytopenia, frequent bone marrow involvement and no peripheral lymphadenopathy. These features differ markedly from those associated with the other subtypes of Hodgkin's disease. Of the four Rye subtypes, however, nodular sclerosis has the most distinctive features. It is undoubtedly the most common subtype found in the mediastinum (Lukes *et al.*,

1966) and occurs most frequently in females, especially those aged 15–34 years (Berard *et al.*, 1971); it is usually associated with a favourable prognosis, a feature which must be related in part to the infrequency with which it progresses to an unfavourable histologic subtype (Strum and Rappaport, 1971b). Despite these differences, nodular sclerosis shares many features in common with the other histologic varieties of Hodgkin's disease. All four subtypes have similar anatomic distributions (Table 2.1) at autopsy (Thomas and Berard, 1973). Although it

Table 2.1 Hodgkin's disease at autopsy (From Thomas, L. B. and Berard, C. W. (1973), by courtesy of *GANN*)

| | Per cent | | | |
Anatomical site	LP	MC	LD	NS
Lymph nodes	81	90	89	88
Spleen	81	84	63	74
Liver	65	61	63	57
Bone	78	76	58	61
Lung and pleura	20	48	53	71
Heart and pericardium	10	10	21	21
Stomach	11	13	16	17
Pancreas	16	26	16	17
Kidneys	16	29	21	17
Adrenal glands	24	22	16	30
Dura and CNS	19	17	0	25
Skin	0	13	5	0

clearly has a predilection for the mediastinum, there is a high incidence of abdominal involvement in nodular sclerosis (Dorfman, 1971) and vascular invasion occurs as frequently as it does with mixed cellularity (Rappaport *et al.*, 1971). Furthermore, nodular sclerosis cannot be viewed as the subtype of the young which is associated with a favourable prognosis. The proportion of Hodgkin's disease occuring in children in countries such as Uganda is higher than in Europe and America (Burn *et al.*, 1971; Davies and Owor, 1965); yet the disease is more aggressive and more malignant subtypes predominate (Olweny *et al.*, 1971): Even in the United States, nodular sclerosis is not uniformly associated with a favourable prognosis, since this feature is apparently limited to females (Thomas and Berard, 1973); One should also realise that this subtype does apparently progress to the lymphocyte depleted stage (Table 2.2) with a greater frequency than has been appreciated in the past (Thomas and Berard, 1973) and it has been stated that if one searches Hodgkin's tissue carefully, a great histologic identity between nodular sclerosis and

Table 2.2 Hodgkin's disease at autopsy (From Thomas, L. B. and Berard, C. W. (1973), by courtesy of *GANN*)

Histology at diagnosis	Total		Histologic progression at autopsy (83 cases)							
			LP		MC		LD sclerotic		LD sarcomatous	
	Male	Female	Male	Female	Male	Female	Male	Female	Male	Female
LP	14	2	1	0	1	2	7	0	5	0
MC	17	4			1	0	12	3	4	1
LD	10	5					0	3	10	2
NS	16	15			1	8	2	2	13	5
Total	57	26	1	0	3	10	21	8	32	8

the other subtypes is observed (Smithers, 1971). It seems clear that each of the Rye subtypes defies simple categorisation based on age, sex or anatomic distribution. Admittedly each histologic variant has certain distinctive features, but they all share certain characteristics in common. Furthermore, different subtypes seem to predominate in various countries (Table 2.3) and it is not clear whether each subtype has a

Table 2.3 Rye subtype distribution of the histologic types of Hodgkin's disease in several countries

| Country | % of histologic types | | | | |
	LP	NS	MC	LD	Total no. of patients
(1) Argentina (Braylan *et al.*, 1973)	13	35	42	8	144
(2) Australia (Hanson, 1964)		15			251
(3) Colombia (Correa and O'Conor, 1971)	17	12	51	22	102
(4) Denmark (Anderson *et al.*, 1970b)	17	32	34	17	142
(5) England (Gough, 1970)	20	15	29	36	96
(6) Finland (Franssila *et al.*, 1967)	9	47	33	11	97
(7) Germany (Hamann *et al.*, 1970)	15	41	21	23	508
(8) Italy (DiPietro and Pizzetti, 1966)		15			100
(9) Peru (Chang, 1967)	40·5	7·9	22·4	29·1	138
(10) South Africa (Selzer *et al.*, 1972)	14	26	35	25	122
(11) Sweden (Landberg and Larsson, 1969)	12	21	54	13	149
(12) Uganda (Olweny *et al.*, 1971)	8	7	47	38	100
(13) USA (Berard *et al.*, 1971)	16	35	33	13	277
(14) USA (Lukes *et al.*, 1966)	16·7	39·5	25·7	18	377
(15) USA (O'Conor *et al.*, 1972)	12·2	40·6	30·3	11·1	389
(16) USA (Strum and Rappaport, 1971a)	12·6	37·8	36	9·5	255

Nodular sclerosis type included, but Rye classification not strictly followed

bimodal age–specific incidence curve. Smithers (1970) observed a bimodal pattern for all subtypes but nodular sclerosis; Stalsberg (1972) observed a bimodality for all four Rye subtypes, but only mixed cellularity possessed this feature in a study conducetd by O'Conor *et al.*, (1972) in the United States. We do not know the meaning of the Rye subtypes but what must be accepted are the facts that this classification relates to prognosis not aetiology and that each subtype has its own distinctive features. Available histologic evidence neither supports nor refutes the concept that Hodgkin's disease is one or more entities. At present it would seem best to focus on specific questions relating to these subtypes. Do they all have bimodal age specific incidence rates? Why does nodular sclerosis involve the mediastinum so frequently and if its favourable prognosis is limited to females, what are the possible explanations for this? Are granulomatous thymomas and nodular sclerosing Hodgkin's disease identical as Nickels *et al.* (1973) have suggested? The answers to these and other questions can not help but provide information about the aetiology of Hodgkin's disease.

Epidemiologic evidence suggesting heterogeneity

International comparisons of the incidence of Hodgkin's disease and analyses of factors such as sex, socio-economic status and urban–rural differences suggest an epidemiologic heterogeneity for different age groups with this disorder. The classical young adult–adult bimodal incidence curve, observed in Western urbanised countries, contrasts sharply with the unimodal (adult peak) curve in Japan and other Asian countries (MacMahon, 1966; Wakasa, 1972). While these different patterns have been interpreted as supporting the concept that Hodgkin's disease might be a different entity in the 15–34 and 50-year and older age groups (MacMahon, 1966), it must be remembered that the Japanese pattern is characterised by low rates in both the childhood and young adult age groups. Furthermore, there are many unusual features of the lymphoreticular malignancies in Japan, ranging from a low incidence of certain other lymphomas to a relatively poor prognosis for Hodgkin's disease in contrast to that in Western countries (Anderson *et al.*, 1970). These peculiarities make clear the need to carefully interpret the Hodgkin's disease pattern in Asian countries. That caution is required is further underlined by the different incidence patterns observed internationally by Correa and O'Conor (1971). This study suggests that incidence rates in childhood are high when those in the young adult group are low. In contrast to Japan, then, the pattern seen in developing countries such as Peru is indicative of a reciprocal relationship between these two age groups. But what is of even greater importance is the fact that the different patterns observed (Correa *et al.*, 1972) are dynamic since each type appears to be related to the stage of economic development of a country. With increasing urbanisation, rates in children decline but increase in young adults. Economic stratification has no apparent effect on the incidence of Hodgkin's disease in the elderly. In the United States, Shimkin (1955) observed an increase in mortality rates from 6·9 to 17·0 per million population between 1925 and 1950 (Figure 2.1). An increase in the mean age at death was also apparent and interestingly,

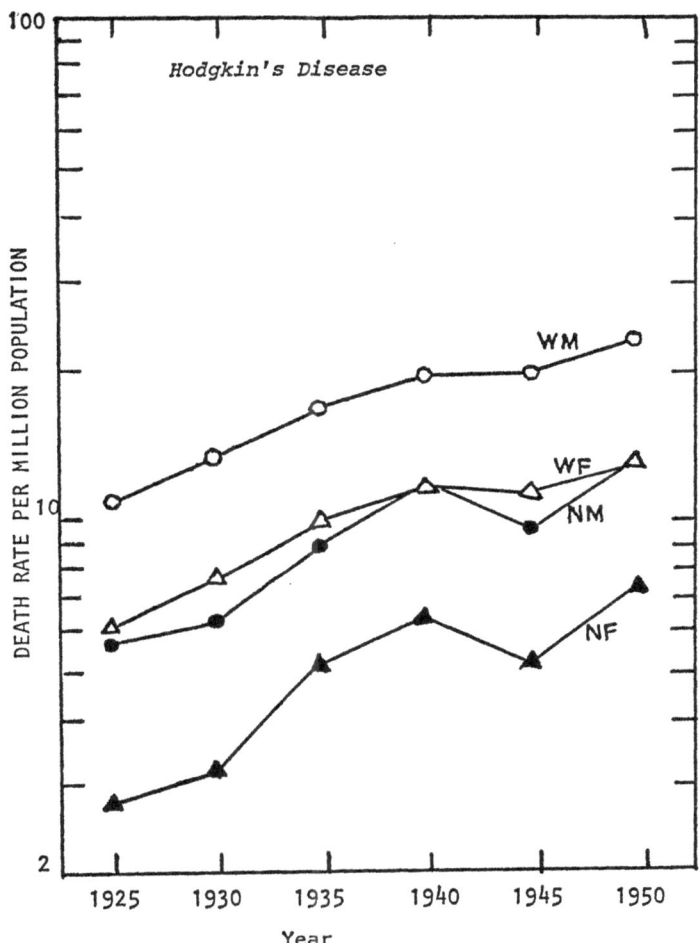

Figure 2.1 Death rate from Hodgkin's disease, by race and sex, United States Death Registration States, 1923–51. WM, white male; WF, white female; NM, non-white male; NF, non-white female. (From Shimkin, M. (1955), by courtesy of *Blood*)

mortality rates declined for those aged 0–14 years but increased for all other age groups. It would seem then that important differences in incidence are apparent for various age groups with this disease, particularly between children and adults.

Differences in sex ratio for various age groups with Hodgkin's disease are also indicative of the heterogeneity within this disorder. MacMahon (1966) refers to five surveys and in four the sex ratio was significantly lower for the 15–34-year age group (sex ratio close to unity) than for those 50 years of age or older (sex ratio, 2:1). Subsequent data, obtained from several tumour registries throughout the world, suggest that this situation is not so clear cut (Doll *et al.*, 1970) and in fact rates for males appear to exceed those for females at all ages. Another study which reviewed data on Hodgkin's disease from Norway, Sweden, Denmark and Finland did not find significant differences in sex ratio between the 15–35 and over 50-year age groups (Stalsberg, 1972). What can be accepted as established with regard to sex ratios in Hodgkin's disease is that this disorder occurs with greater frequency in males, regardless of the age incidence pattern in a country. This is true in countries with classical bimodal incidence curves (MacMahon, 1966), in Japan with its unimodal pattern (Wakasa, 1972) and in South American countries with childhood and adult age peaks (Correa and O'Conor, 1971). Furthermore, male predominance appears to be most marked in the childhood age groups (Solidoro *et al.*, 1966; Jelliffe and Thompson, 1955; Newall, 1965). In a study of 1484 deaths due to this disorder in patients less than 20 years of age, Miller (1966) found that males comprised 76 per cent of all cases among white children, aged 5–11 years. This proportion decreased to 60 per cent for the 11–19-year age group. These observations suggest that the greatest differences in sex ratio exist between the 0–14 and older age groups. In Uganda, with its unusual lymphoma pattern, a high sex ratio is limited to the first two decades of life (Wright, 1972). Similar observations have been made in Latin America with a high incidence of childhood Hodgkin's disease (Correa, 1972).

Socio-economic factors appear to be closely bound to variations in incidence and sex ratio in Hodgkin's disease. But in view of the many differences observed, it is essential to consider the importance of this factor for various age groups with this disorder. In Western, urbanised countries such as England and Wales, evidence has been presented which suggests that the highest social class has the highest risk of Hodgkin's disease (MacMahon, 1966). However, two subsequent investigations in the same country failed to confirm this association (Registrar General's Decennial Supplement, 1971; Alderson and Nayak, 1972). In upstate New York, mortality rates for males residing in high socio-economic counties were only slightly higher than the overall adult rate for this disorder (Vianna *et al.*, 1974a). In sharp contrast to these conflicting observations on a national and regional level, international comparisons suggest that social factors might exert their greatest influence on the incidence of childhood and young adult age groups of

Hodgkin's disease. This is clearly suggested by the reciprocal relationship between these two age groups observed by Correa and O'Conor (1971). But the impact of social and economic factors goes beyond influencing age–specific incidence patterns. Where the incidence of childhood Hodgkin's disease is high, this is due to high rates in males; not just males, but males with poor histologic subtypes (Correa and O'Conor, 1971). In contrast nodular sclerosis is more prevalent in wealthy urbanised countries which are characterised by a young adult age peak. Socio-economic factors might also explain the impressive urban–rural differences observed in certain countries. In urban Norway, Hodgkin's disease has young adult and adult age peaks whereas in rural areas the pattern is characterised by incidence rates which are somewhat higher in male children but lower in young adult males (Correa and O'Conor, 1971). Dörken and Singer-Bakker (1972) found a small but distinct prevalence of Hodgkin's disease for male cases under 30 years of age in rural regions of Northern Germany and Fasal *et al.* (1968) found high incidence and mortality rates among young male farm residents in California. It will be interesting to see if this intermediate pattern shifts to the classical bimodal incidence curve in areas of this type as urbanisation occurs.

The epidemiologic and histologic evidence presented here and in Chapter 1, leaves us with several important concepts. Environmental factors undoubtedly play a major role in the aetiology of Hodgkin's disease. It is a dynamic disorder characterised by different incidence patterns internationally and regionally, especially when factors such as age, sex and urban–rural differences are examined. There are many features which suggest heterogeneity within this disease, especially when childhood and adult age groups are compared. There is at present one factor which appears to underline the differences observed in age–specific incidence, sex ratio, geographic distribution and histologic subtype—the socio-economic stratification of the communities studied. It must be realised that rate and degree of urbanisation undoubtedly varies in different areas; so too should the patterns of Hodgkin's disease. But we now are in a position to ask a rather specific question: based on what we know of the environmental world, what types of factors are capable of inducing the changes observed?

EPIDEMIOLOGIC PROBES

Although epidemiologic data supports the concept that real differences exist between childhood and adult Hodgkin's disease, we clearly do not know the nature of this heterogeneity. New avenues of approach are requied to further our understanding of this admittedly complex problem. Of the many possibilities, there are four probes which can be used to evaluate Hodgkin's disease in these two age groups for additional differences. In 1971, it was hypothesised that prior tonsillectomy might act as a predisposing factor to this disorder in individuals 40 years of age or less (Vianna *et al.*, 1971a). This case–general population control study suggested that prior tonsillectomy increased the risk of developing Hodgkin's disease by a factor of 2·9 (Table 2.4). However

Table 2.4 History of tonsillectomy among Hodgkin's and control patients aged 6–40. Nassau and Suffolk counties, NY, 1960–69

Group	Hodgkin's disease	Controls
Total patients	109	109
Total status known	101	107
Tonsillectomy: Yes	67	43
No	34	64
Relative odds $\dfrac{67 \times 64}{34 \times 43} = 2\text{·}9$		

it is important to realise that less than 10 per cent of the patients studied were under 15 years of age at diagnosis. Obviously little can be said about the possible effect of prior tonsillectomy in this age group, but this matter should be considered. Large numbers of cases may well be required to conduct a tonsillectomy study in childhood Hodgkin's disease, since many cases and controls might be too young to have had this operation. It is also important to realise that there is no evidence suggesting that the age at tonsillectomy differs for cases and sib controls, the mean age in both groups being around 7 years (Vianna *et al.*, 1974a). It would be unlikely therefore that any differences observed would be attributable to this factor. The tonsillectomy hypothesis will be dealt with in detail later in this chapter.

Evaluation of different age groups with Hodgkin's disease for seasonality represents another important epidemiologic probe. Analysis of months of birth in childhood and adult age groups might be particularly informative since this is usually indicative of some natal and/or prenatal influence. Fraumeni and Li (1969) found a significant excess of male children, aged 15 years or less at death, born during July and August. Bjelke (1969) detected no significant seasonal variation in birth months for cases of Hodgkin's disease of all ages, and Bailar and Gurian (1964) reported negative results for the lymphomas as a group. Thus, this matter is not resolved and it will be important to consider age, sex and urban–rural factors in future studies.

Other studies have evaluated the question of seasonality in Hodgkin's disease by month of onset. Cridland (1961) reported a peak in seasonal onset of Hodgkin's disease during the months of December and January. Month of onset was defined in this study as the first appearance of peripheral node enlargement and no evidence of generalised disease within six months after onset. Using the same criteria, Innes and Newall (1961) found that 41 per cent of their cases had onsets between January and March. However, it was pointed out that both studies were quite selective in the cases employed and a seasonal variation in the onset of symptoms probably relates to perception and diagnosis rather than to aetiologic factors (MacMahon, 1966). Furthermore, studies in Norway (Bjelke, 1969), Israel (Meytes and Modan, 1969) and nine metropolitan areas of the United States (Newell, 1972) failed to detect a seasonal tendency when the patients studied were not restricted to those with localised disease. In sharp contrast to these results, several reports from Germany suggest that there is a peak in the clinical onset of Hodgkin's disease during the winter months. Uhl *et al.* (1967) found a peak during the winter months when the first manifestation of disease was used as the determinant of month of onset. Hartwich and Schlabeck (1970) and Dörken and Singer-Bakker (1972) also found a marked excess of cases during the winter months, with a peak in January and a deficit during the summer months. Another study (Fraumeni and Li, 1969), dealing only with childhood Hodgkin's disease in the United States, suggested that more than the expected number of cases have their clinical onsets in December. To date then, the possibility that there is a seasonality by month of onset in Hodgkin's disease remains unsettled. It is imperative, however, that future studies examine this question for different age groups.

It seems clear that antigens of the human histocompatibility system (HL–A) can modulate certain diseases. Since Amiel (1967) first reported an association between Hodgkin's disease and 4c antigens (HL–A5, W5, W18 and W15), several studies have confirmed this observation (Forbes and Morris, 1970; Zervas *et al.*, 1970; Bodmer, 1972). Others (Kissmeyer-Nielsen *et al.*, 1971; Falk and Osoba, 1971) have observed significant associations with HL–A1 and HL–A8 antigens, but this requires further evaluation. Falk and Osoba (1971) also suggested that the HL–A1 and HL–A8 antigens are frequently associated with the lymphocyte predominant and mixed cellularity subtypes of Hodgkin's disease, whereas patients with nodular sclerosis have an increased frequency of HL–A5. In a study of HL–A anitgens in patients with Hodgkin's disease and unaffected family members, Forbes and Morris (1972) presented evidence that relevant antigens were present before the disease developed for in six cases where a patient was found to be W5 positive, the antigen was also found to be present on a parent's lymphocytes. It was further suggested that certain patients develop Hodgkin's disease because of a genetically determined predisposition which could control immune responsiveness. Using HL–A typing, it will be important to determine the antigen distribution of different age groups with this disorder regionally and internationally.

Other markers which might be used to evaluate the heterogeneity within Hodgkin's disease are the two tumour associated antigens, the F (fast) and S (slow) antigens, which have been found in diseased spleens and lymph nodes (Order *et al.*, 1972; Chism *et al.*, 1973). This probe is limited somewhat by the facts that the antigens are not specific for Hodgkin's disease and at present a serologic assay is not available. However, the S and F antigens are found in much higher amounts in Hodgkin's disease tissue and it is possible that varying concentrations might be found in different age groups and histologic subtypes.

The four approaches mentioned by no means exhaust the available tools for evaluating the heterogeneity within Hodgkin's disease. Others (Piperno and Kaller, 1973) have examined the DNA-dependent DNA polymerase activities of various subtypes of Hodgkin's disease and found that the nodular sclerosis and mixed-cellularity forms can be distinguished from one another and control polymerases. But as our knowledge increases and additional differences are detected, we must constantly consider whether these observations can be related holistically or not.

POSSIBLE INFECTIOUS AETIOLOGY IN HODGKIN'S DISEASE

The possibility that Hodgkin's disease might be infectious in nature is by no means a new hypothesis. Admittedly epidemiology can never prove or disprove this proposition, but it can determine whether this disorder possesses characteristics which are compatible with this concept. It is important to realise at the onset that none of the descriptive epidemiologic features of Hodgkin's disease is inconsistent with an infectious aetiology. Indeed there are many examples of acute infectious diseases in which variations in time and place, age shifts and changes in sex ratios have occurred. Social factors can clearly influence the incidence patterns of certain infectious diseases, as well as their clinical and histologic picture. While some might argue that the age distribution of Hodgkin's disease is inconsistent with an infectious aetiology, to the contrary, bimodality has been observed in disorders such as tuberculosis. But to stop at this point is not acceptable. Specific questions must be asked upon which other studies might be based and laboratory hypothesis tested. As mentioned earlier in this chapter, evidence has been presented which suggests that prior tonsillectomy might be a predisposing factor to Hodgkin's disease in young adults (Vianna *et al.*, 1971a). This hypothesis has been evaluated in several subsequent reports and although results have been somewhat conflicting, this might be due in part to the different approaches taken and age groups studied. Ruuskanen *et al.* (1971) studied fifty-three patients of all ages in Finland and failed to confirm this observation. In another non-geographic based study, Johnson and Johnson (1972) interpreted their data as not supporting the tonsillectomy hypothesis. This study was the first to use sibs as controls for Hodgkin's disease patients. Although the use of sibs undoubtedly represents a good socio-economic control group, it is important to realise that sibs are likely to have similar tonsillectomy histories. Despite this obvious bias against the hypothesis re-evaluation of the Johnsons' data (Cole *et al.*, 1973; Pike and Smith, 1973; Shimaoka *et al.*, 1973) indicated that the relative risk was 2·1 which is consistent with the estimated relative risk of 2·9 observed in the Long Island case–general population control study (Vianna *et al.*, 1971b). Another hospital based study of all cancers found a significant association only between prior tonsillectomy and thyroid cancer and Hodgkin's disease (Bross *et al.*, 1971). Newell *et al.* (1973) found no significant difference in tonsillectomy histories between cases and matched sib controls, but this report considered only live patients whose physicians granted permission to be interviewed. The most recent case-sib control study (Vianna *et al.*, 1974a) of Hodgkin's disease in patients 40 years of age or less in upstate New York, suggested that the relative risk of prior tonsillectomy was 2·0. This study provided further evidence that sibs are likely to have similar tonsillectomy histories (thereby biasing against the tonsillectomy hypothesis), that future studies should be area based, and specific age groups and live and dead cases should be considered. Suffice it to say that there is sufficient evidence supporting the tonsillectomy hypothesis to make it a high priority for future epidemiologic study. If this proposition is confirmed, the virologist can ask what oncogenic viruses,

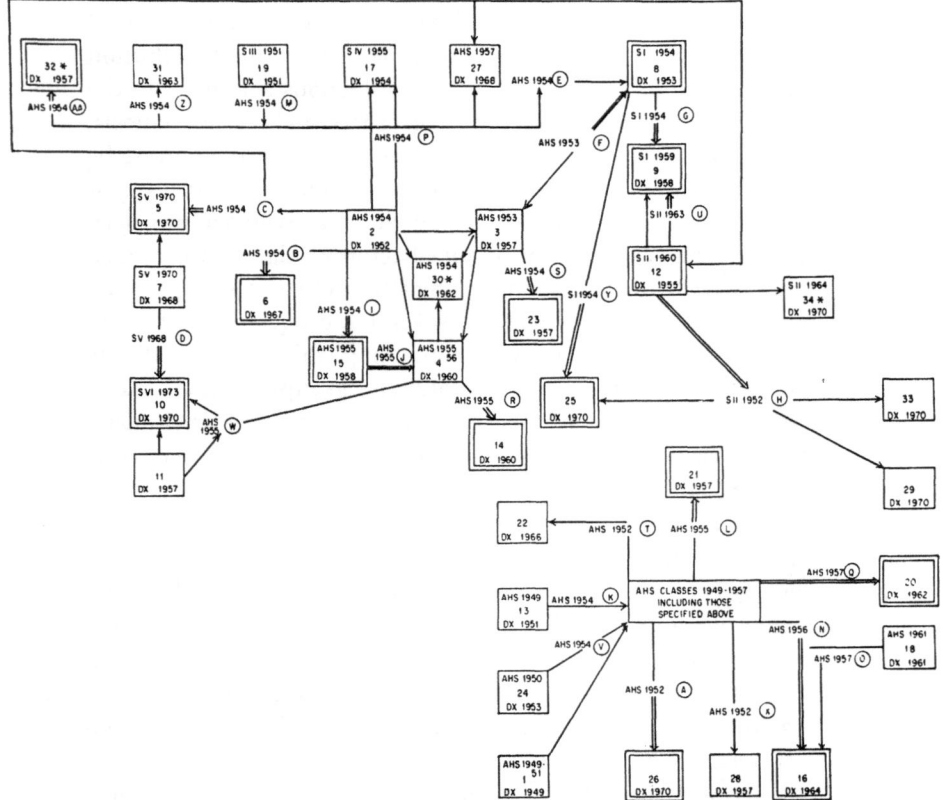

Figure 2.2 Interrelationships between lymphoma cases and contacts in Albany, NY. Numbers = cases; Letters = contacts; Double-lined boxes = case and contact lived in same house before diagnosis; * = lymphoma other than Hodgkin's disease. (From Vianna, N.J. *et al.* (1972), by courtesy of *Ann. Int.Med.*)

with tropism to lymphoreticular tissue, do the tonsils act as an immunologic barrier against?

If Hodgkin's disease is to be viewed hypothetically as an infectious disorder, another specific question is whether transmission occurs. The strongest suggestion of horizontal transmission in man comes from studies of groupings with this disorder. The three groups of Hodgkin's disease described in upstate New York had several characteristics in common (Vianna *et al.*, 1971b; Vianna *et al.*, 1972):

(1) Case-to-case contact was unusual; the majority of cases were associated through some healthy intermediary. This becomes apparent in the Albany grouping when it is realised that the starting point for this investigation centred around three directly linked cases (cases 2, 3 and 4—Figure 2.2). If we exclude these links and those involving patients with other lymphomas, there were only three case–to–case associations among the thirty-one linked cases with Hodgkin's disease.

(2) Although all of these groupings were school based, elementary schools were not involved. In Albany (Figure 2.2) and downstate (Figure 2.3), most of the cases were high school students whereas the upstate grouping (Figure 2.4) centred around a medical college.

(3) In each group, there was a core of students who knew each other before Hodgkin's disease was diagnosed in any of them. Although all age groups were represented, most of the cases were young and none was under the age of 14 years. In considering the upstate New York groupings and those reported by Dworsky and Henderson (1974) and Klinger and Minton (1973), the age of cases ranged from 14 to 74 years and forty-three of the fifty-five cases were under 40 years of age at diagnosis. It should be realised that none of these studies was conducted in a manner that would exclude younger cases of Hodgkin's disease. This observation strengthens the concept of heterogeneity between the childhood and adult age groups.

(4) No predominant pattern with respect to sex was observed among linked cases.

(5) All of the Rye subtypes were observed in both young and old patients. In the Albany group (Vianna *et al.*, 1972) no significant difference in subtype was observed when the age of patients was tabulated.

(6) There were many instances where a student, who attended the same class as a case remained in good health but Hodgkin's disease

developed in another member of the family, usually an adult living in the same household. In Albany (Figure 2.2), of the fifteen linked cases outside the school system, nine lived in the same household with a school-age contact who had a specific relationship with at least one school-based case. The important point here is that none of the individuals involved in the case–intermediary–case pattern was related transiently.

(7) Where it was possible to follow the subsequent time–place associations of an individual (case or contact) involved in one of the upstate New York groupings, these individuals associated with other people from different areas, some of whom eventually developed Hodgkin's disease. In the Albany group (Figure 2.2), contact H, the

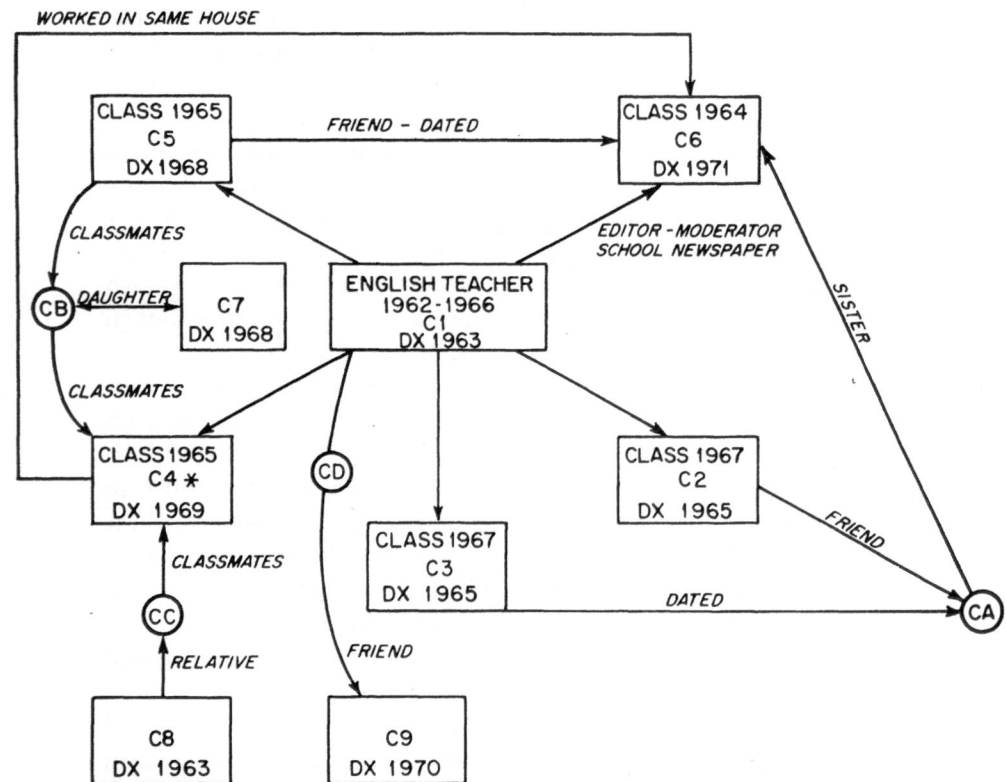

Figure 2.3 Interrelationships between lymphoma cases and contacts in downstate New York. Patients with lymphoma are indicated by the numbers C1 through C9. The letters indicate contacts. DX = diagnosis; * = lymphoma other than Hodgkin's disease. (From Vianna, N. J. *et al.* (1972), by courtesy of *Ann. Int. Med.*)

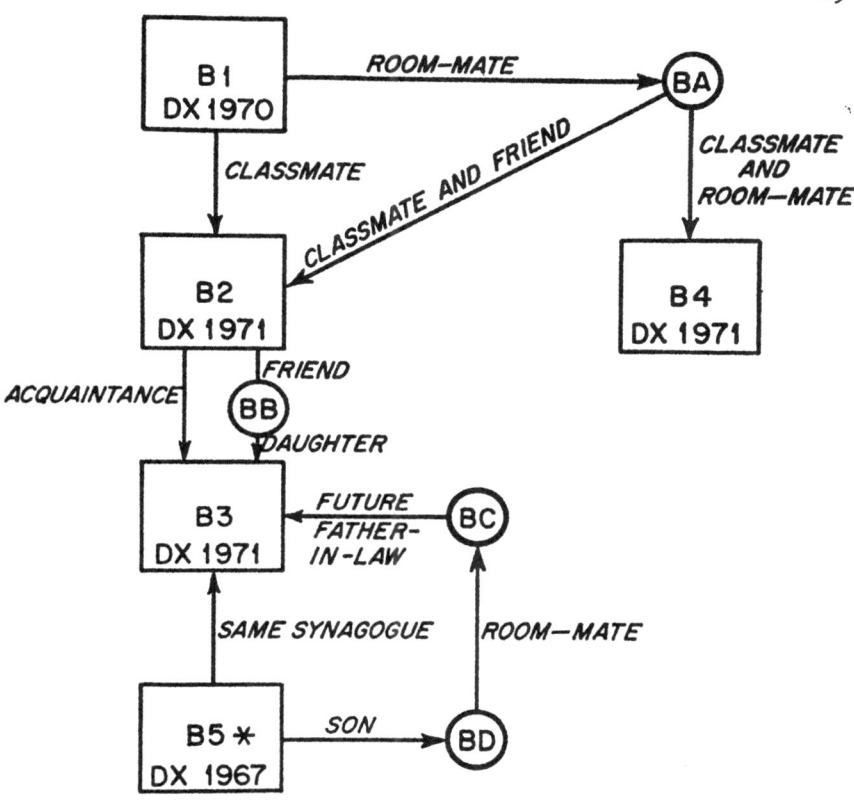

Figure 2.4 Interrelationships between lymphoma cases and contacts in upstate New York. B1 through B5 indicate patients with lymphoma; BA, BB, BC, and BD are contacts. DX = diagnosis; * = lymphoma other than Hodgkin's disease. (From Vianna, N.J. *et al.* (1972), by courtesy of *Ann. Int. Med.*)

sister of case 12, was a close friend of case 8 and other cases during her high school days. This girl remains in good health up to the present but the disease developed in cases 25, 29 and 33, all of whom worked with her in two different banks in an area outside of Albany, several years after she graduated from school. Case 2, one of the index cases, was closely associated with several student cases and healthy contacts during his high school days. After graduating he attended a university in a different county of upstate New York and joined a fraternity. Another student who belonged to the same club subsequently developed Hodgkin's disease and the father of case 2 was diagnosed with lymphosarcoma. Case 31 worked in a summer camp in close association with a healthy student who was a high school classmate of case 2. Case 31 subsequently attended a university in another state and was a room-mate of a girl from yet another state. After graduation, case 31 went to Europe where she developed Hodgkin's disease in 1963. Her room-mate remained in the United States where she was diagnosed with Hodgkin's disease shortly thereafter. In the upstate grouping (Figure 2.4) a similar situation involved contact A. This girl was a room-mate of case B1 while in an upstate medical school but subsequently transferred to a university in Florida where she was both a room-mate and classmate of case B4 who was diagnosed with Hodgkin's disease in 1971. These secondary groupings had all of the features of those in Albany, upstate and downstate, including a specific and close association between cases and/or intermediaries.

(8) Using dates of diagnosis, the mean time interval between cases was around three years. It is important to realise that none of the Hodgkin's disease groupings was the result of formal attempts to establish time–space clustering.

Since the Albany grouping was the largest of its kind, both in the number of associated cases and the time period during which these events apparently occurred, annual rates for Hodgkin's disease between 1950 and 1970 (Figure 2.5) were evaluated. The major question was whether the trend for this disease, over the twenty-one year period during which thirty-one cases of Hodgkin's disease were linked, was suggestive of an epidemic period? The average annual incidence for the 208 histologically confirmed cases among residents of this area was 3·7 per 100 000 per annum (Vianna *et al.*, 1972). From 1950 through 1952, yearly rates were below this average, but remained above it from 1953 through 1961 (Figure 2.5). Peak years during this period were 1958 and 1961 with rates of 5·6 and 5·8 per 100 000 population respectively. There was a dramatic fall in rates from 1962 through 1965 with further peaks in 1966 and 1967. A comparison of the average incidence rates during the period of high rates, 1953 through 1959, and the following period 1963 through 1969, revealed a statistically significant difference in rates between these two periods. In addition when the Albany County case rates were compared with those for the rest of upstate New York, they were significantly higher during the period 1953 through 1959 and lower during the 1963 through 1969 period. These observations were suggestive of an epidemic period in the county followed by a period of relative community immunity. In addition, the mean age of cases during the 1953 through 1959 period was lower than that for the rest of upstate New York and was significantly higher from 1963 through 1969. Both this shift to an older age group and the apparent epidemic curve were compatible with the possibility that Hodgkin's disease was acting as an infectious disease in the community.

If the epidemiologic characteristics suggested by the tonsillectomy hypothesis are merged with those derived from the Hodgkin's groups, our search for a hypothetical aetiologic agent centres around a virus with the following features: oncogenic potential, probable lymphotropism, possible inactivation by immunocompetent tonsillar tissue, prolonged latency, an asymptomatic carrier state and community immunity with a shift to an older age group. Needless to say, all of these considerations are hypothetical. A major limitation to the evaluation of the Hodgkin's disease groups described was that the statistical significance of the case linkages observed could not be determined (Vianna *et al.*, 1972; *Brit. Med. J.*, editorial, 1972). But detailed analysis of those characteristics which all of the Hodgkin's disease groups had in common did provide the information required for designing a more objective study. The downstate New York grouping served as the exempler for this investigation since it was well-circumscribed and yet all of the characteristics previously mentioned are present (Figure 2.3). This grouping centred around a high school with 1000 students who were divided into 40 classes of 25 students each. The index case, case C1 joined the faculty in September 1962. As one of six English teachers, she taught only certain classes in the years 1962 through 1966. All of the students who developed Hodgkin's disease in the school, in fact in the whole town, from 1960 through 1970 had several things in common:

(1) They were all closely associated prior to and during the time this teacher attended school, as well as after she died.

(2) They all had tutorial contact with this teacher, despite the fact that most of them were in different classes.

(3) There was apparent transmission to household contacts (case C7 and C9 were adults who resided in the same house as a healthy student who attends the same classes as a student case).

The most obvious features of this configuration of cases was that at a point in time an index case enters the school setting, apparently coming into varying degrees of contact with many students while she has Hodgkin's disease. During the following years several secondary cases occurred among members of the student body. This index–secondary case approach was used to test the hypothesis that in the 777 public schools of all types in Nassau and Suffolk Counties, New York, where a case of Hodgkin's disease occurred in a teacher or student, more than the expected number of additional cases would occur among teachers, students or both. Two objective methods were used to test this hypothesis (Vianna and Polan, 1973). One was to determine whether high schools with at least one case who was both diagnosed and stayed in that institution for at least one year from 1960 through 1964 were more likely to have additional cases from 1965 through 1969 than matched schools without cases during the earlier period. The results of this two time period approach indicated that of the eight schools with cases in the earlier period, five had additional cases in the latter period (Table 2.5). Matched control schools had no cases during the years 1965–69.

Table 2.5   Two time period distribution of public high schools with cases of Hodgkin's disease, their matched controls and schools of comparable size in Nassau–Suffolk counties, New York (Reprinted, by courtesy of *New Eng. J. Med.*, **289**:499, 1973)

	1965–69		
1960–64	*Schools with cases*	*Schools with no cases*	*Totals*
Schools with cases	5	3	8
Matched controls—no cases	0	16	16
All comparable schools—no cases	6	137	143

When all other public high schools of similar size were contrasted with case schools, only 4·2 per cent of these schools (6 out of 143) had cases during the period 1965–69. All analyses showed highly significant differences. The other approach was to analyse specific schools with respect to individual cases. In schools with index cases, one might expect to observe greater than the expected number of secondary cases. Index cases were predefined as the first case (teacher or student) diagnosed with the disease while in a given school. To be considered an index case, the patient also had to stay in the school for at least one year after diagnosis. The rationale for including this factor was fourfold:

(1) In all of the groups previously described, there was the opportunity for multiple contacts in addition to those documented.

(2) In the downstate grouping, the teacher–index case remained in school several years after diagnosis.

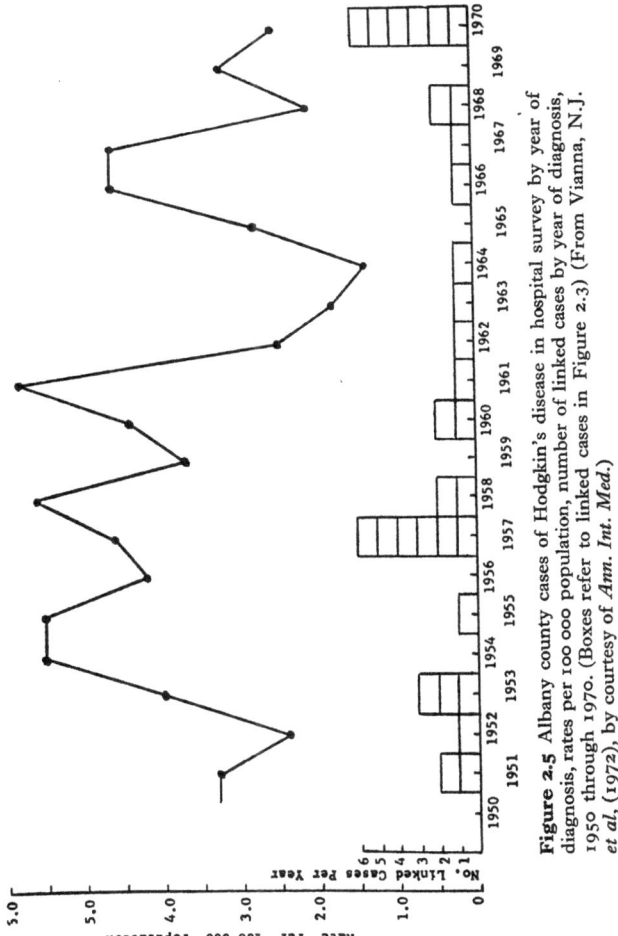

Figure 2.5 Albany county cases of Hodgkin's disease in hospital survey by year of diagnosis, rates per 100 000 population, number of linked cases by year of diagnosis, 1950 through 1970. (Boxes refer to linked cases in Figure 2.3) (From Vianna, N.J. *et al*, (1972), by courtesy of *Ann. Int. Med.*)

Lymphoreticular malignancies

(3) The decision to limit links between cases to one single intermediary was arbitrary. The possibility that several intermediaries might in fact be required was therefore not excluded (e.g. case–contact–contact–case).

(4) The possibility that host factors might be important in Hodgkin's disease had to be considered.

Table 2.6 Cases of Hodgkin's disease observed in Nassau–Suffolk County Public Schools with index cases (1960–70) (Reprinted, by courtesy of *New Eng. J. Med.*, **289**:499–502 (September 6), 1973)

Type of school	Index* Student	Teacher	Secondary* Student	Teacher	Non associated* Student
High†:					
A		62 M-1962	16 F-1967		
B	17 F-1960		15 M-1964	60 M-1962	
			22 F-1964	34 M-1964	
			18 F-1966	40 M-1970	
			22 F-1969		
			21 M-1970		
C	15 F-1968			36 M-1969	
D‡	10 M-1962				
E	17 M-1964		19 M-1964		
F	17 M-1966		16 M-1967		
G	10 M-1962		14 M-1968		18 F-1962
H	11 M-1969				
I	15 M-1968		20 M-1969		
J		31 M-1960	15 F-1966	36 M-1967	
			18 M-1967	35 M-1969	
			26 F-1969		
K	16 M-1964			53 M-1968	
L	17 F-1969				
M	16 F-1967				
N	14 F-1963				
College:					
O	17 M-1966		22 M-1966		25 F-1969
			20 M-1967		
			18 M-1968		
P	20 M-1964		23 M-1969		
			22 M-1969		
Q§	16 F-1960		20 F-1962		19 M-1967
			21 M-1963		
Elementary:					
R		16 F-1960	9 F-1967		
S	8 M-1960				
T	8 M-1965				

* Age, sex and year of diagnosis   † Junior and senior
‡ Same index case as G   § Same index case as R

If transmission does occur, it might be necessary for a case to be associated with many individuals before a susceptible host is found. Secondary cases were defined as those who were present in the same school for at least one year while the index patient was present and were diagnosed at a later date than the index case. Establishing contact with the index case, either direct or indirect, was not a prerequisite. Non-associated cases were those who were diagnosed at a later time than the index case but not present in the same school during an overlapping period with either the index case or a secondary case. This type of case was excluded from all statistical analysis. The index, secondary and non-associated cases identified in this study are listed in Table 2.6. The number of cases observed in schools with index cases was significantly higher than the expected number of cases as were case rates for students and teachers (Table 2.7). Thus, both approaches suggested

Table 2.7 Rates for secondary cases of Hodgkin's disease among students and teachers in Nassau–Suffolk Public Schools with index cases according to type of institution (1960–70) (Reprinted, by courtesy of *New Eng. J. Med.*, **289**:499–502 (September 6), 1973)

Type of school	No. of schools with index case	Persons counted through 1970	Person year	No. of secondary cases	Rate*
Students					
Elementary	3	2541	20 363	1	4·9
High	14	28 369	172 076	13	7·6
College	3	12 277	76 818	7	9·1
All types	20	43 817	269 257	21	7·8
Teachers					
Elementary	3	302	1771	0	0·0
High	14	2729	13 441	7	52·1
College	3	1621	6234	0	0·0
All types	20	4652	21 446	7	32·6

* Rate per 100 000 person year

that some form of transmission might be important in Hodgkin's disease. But it must be emphasised that only 10 per cent of the cases that occurred in the study area between 1960 and 1970 were included in this study. This is due to the fact that each approach considered only public schools with index cases. Private schools were not included in the study. Consequently nothing can be said with regard to all school aged cases nor about cases in the general community (Vianna and Polan, 1973).

There were several additional observations made in the above study. The mean interval between cases for those schools with index cases and at least one secondary case was 3·8 years (median 3 years). This is quite similar to the mean interval between cases observed in the Albany group (Vianna *et al.*, 1972). Furthermore, Hodgkin's disease rates were highest for high schools with the largest teacher and student enrolments (23·8 per 100 000 for schools with a total enrolment of 1500 or greater; 5·3 per 100 000 for those with smaller institutions). This observation is consistent with the suggestion made previously, that for apparent transmission to occur, a case might have to come in contact with a large number of individuals before a susceptible one is found.

The major criticism of this study was that the average annual incidence rate was 1·9 per 100 000 population, which is lower than the average national rate (Pike *et al.*, 1974). However, regional differences in Hodgkin's disease rates have been observed in the United States (Cole *et al.*, 1968; Fraumeni and Li, 1969) and other countries (Wakasa, 1972; Correa and O'Conor, 1971; MacMahon, 1966). Furthermore, while underascertainment of cases could undoubtedly have an effect on the two time period approach, it is unlikely to have significant influence on the results of the index–secondary case approach.

An important question, not included in the teacher–student study (Vianna and Polan, 1973) is whether the cases identified could be related with one another? Recently an attempt was made to determine the number of cases that could be linked directly to other cases, be they teachers or students. Only two index cases could be directly associated with other cases of Hodgkin's disease; both were students, one from high school B, the other from college P (Table 2.6) and they were friends several years before either developed this disorder (Figure 2.6). The index case from school P was also close friends with both student secondary cases in that institution, while they attended high school and college. They all developed Hodgkin's disease in college (Figure 2.6). In contrast the 17-year-old index case (school B) could not be directly associated with other cases. Interestingly three of the secondary cases in school B, including one teacher, could be associated with one another. Thus, of the forty-nine cases (index or secondary) of Hodgkin's disease studied, only seven could be related directly to another case. One additional point is that the case–case associations observed in school B were of an intensity similar to that observed for cases 2, 3 and 4 in the Albany

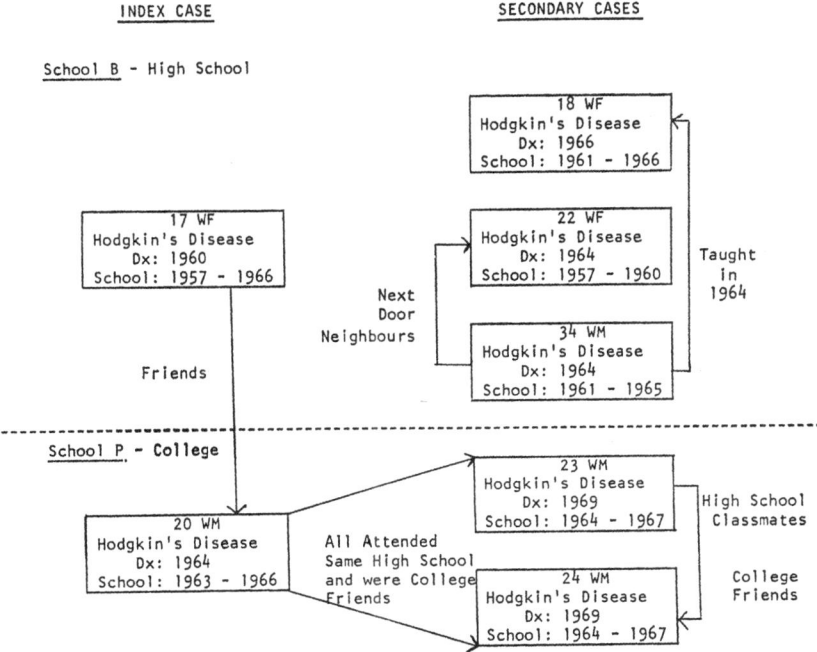

INDEX CASE   SECONDARY CASES

School B - High School

18 WF
Hodgkin's Disease
Dx: 1966
School: 1961 - 1966

17 WF
Hodgkin's Disease
Dx: 1960
School: 1957 - 1966

22 WF
Hodgkin's Disease
Dx: 1964
School: 1957 - 1960

Taught
in
1964

Next
Door
Neighbours

34 WM
Hodgkin's Disease
Dx: 1964
School: 1961 - 1965

Friends

School P. - College

20 WM
Hodgkin's Disease
Dx: 1964
School: 1963 - 1966

23 WM
Hodgkin's Disease
Dx: 1969
School: 1964 - 1967

High School
Classmates

All Attended
Same High School
and were College
Friends

24 WM
Hodgkin's Disease
Dx: 1969
School: 1964 - 1967

College
Friends

Figure 2.6 Associations between Hodgkin's disease cases in two schools in Nassau and Suffolk counties, New York

group (Figure 2.2). Interestingly both groups were the largest observed in their respective studies (Vianna *et al.*, 1972; Vianna and Polan, 1973). While these observations are admittedly based on anecdotal information, they do suggest that the magnitude of a hypothetical outbreak of Hodgkin's disease might be related to the presence of several inter-related cases which act as a continuous source in a given area.

Finally, while most of the Hodgkin's disease groups described have centred around schools, groupings in other settings have been reported. In California seven cases of histologically confirmed Hodgkin's disease occurred among a group of heroin addicts (Dworsky and Henderson, 1974). Although these cases were not linked directly with each other, six of them lived in close proximity. The age of patients ranged from 21 to 43 years of age and both favourable and unfavourable histologic subtypes were observed.

What additional avenues of approach are available for evaluating the transmission hypothesis in Hodgkin's disease? A reasonable extension of the Nassau–Suffolk teacher-student study would be to test the hypothesis that the rate for school teachers might be high. The results of a mortality study of male teachers, 20 years of age and older, dying of this disease in Washington State were recently reported by Milham (1974). Using proportionate mortality analysis, the observed number of teacher deaths due to Hodgkin's disease was significantly greater than the number expected (Table 2.8). The study was interpreted as lending indirect support to the hypothesis that Hodgkin's disease may be horizontally transmitted. While this consideration is important and worthy of further evaluation, it must be emphasised that if teachers do not have significantly higher rates than expected, the Nassau–Suffolk transmission hypothesis is not refuted. The important question that this study raises (Vianna and Polan, 1973) is not what is the rate for Hodgkin's disease among teachers but rather what is the rate for this disorder in schools where an index case was present? This distinction is absolutely essential

Table 2.8 Proportionate mortality analysis* for school-teachers dying of Hodgkin's disease (HD) Washington State male resident deaths, 20 years of age and over. 1950–71 (Reprinted, by courtesy of *New Eng. J. Med.*, **290**:1329, 1974)

Age of death	Proportion of deaths from HD for all occupations	No. of schoolteacher deaths		
			HD	
Year		All causes	observed	expected
20–24	0·0128	16	0	0·20
25–29	0·0142	43	3	0·61
30–34	0·0130	35	1	0·45
35–39	0·0113	38	2	0·43
40–44	0·0081	60	2	0·48
45–49	0·0042	89	0	0·37
50–54	0·0039	131	0	0·51
55–59	0·0031	132	1	0·54
60–64	0·0021	174	1	0·36
65–69	0·0016	160	1	0·26
70–74	0·0016	197	0	0·32
75–79	0·0008	213	1	0·17
80–84	0·0004	185	0	0·07
85*	0·0005	225	0	0·11
Totals		1698	12	4·88

$$* \frac{100 \times \text{observed deaths}}{\text{expected deaths}} = \frac{100 \times 12}{4.88} = 246$$

as evidenced by the fact that the observed rate for teachers in index schools was 32·6, which contrasts with an annual incidence rate for all teachers in the counties studied of 4·3 per 100 000 teacher years, which is similar to the expected rate (Vianna and Polan, 1973).

Another hypothesis worthy of evaluation is that medical personnel, such as physicians might have a higher than expected rate of Hodgkin's disease. Since Hodgkin's disease might occur with greater frequency among members of high socio-economic class and physicians generally belong to this class, their mortality rate must be compared with that for other individuals in this category. In upstate New York, from 1960 through 1972, thirteen male physicians died of Hodgkin's disease (Vianna *et al.*, 1974) a rate of 6·9 per 100 000 per year (Table 2.9).

Table 2.9 **Deaths from Hodgkin's disease among male physicians, 25-years of age and other groups of the same age and sex in upstate New York from 1960–71** (From, Vianna, N. J., Polan, A. K., Keogh, M. *et al.*, by courtesy of *Lancet*, 1974b, in press)

	Hodgkin's disease*	
	Number of deaths	Rate†
Physicians	13	6·90
Upstate New York	1288	3·83
Four selected counties‡	537	4·08

* International classification of diseases, 8th revision, No. 201
† Rate per 100 000 population
‡ Monroe, Nassau, Suffolk and Westchester counties

The comparable rate for males, 25 years of age and over for the same period was 3·83 per 100 000. The difference between these two rates was statistically significant ($p < 0.01$) and the magnitude of increased risk for physicians was 1·8. When the four large counties with the highest median income in upstate New York were considered, the mortality rate was 4·08 per 100 000 which was also significantly different from the rate for physicians ($p < 0.04$). It is interesting that none of the physicians studied were oncologists (Table 2.10). While it is possible that this subspecialty is sufficiently small that one case might not be expected to occur during the thirteen-year study period, one can speculate that if direct contact with a case were alone sufficient for apparent transmission and clinical disease, oncologists should have an exceedingly high risk.

Table 2.10 Subspecialties of thirteen physicians dying of Hodgkin's disease in upstate New York from 1960-72 (From Vianna, N. J., Polan, A. K., Keogh, M. *et al.*, by courtesy of *Lancet*, 1974b, in press)

Subspecialty	Hodgkin's disease
Roentgenology	1
Anaesthesiology	1
General surgery	3
Otolaryngology	1
Neurosurgery	1
General practice	1
Internal medicine	2
Psychiatry	1
Not stated	2

It seems quite likely then that other factors (e.g. alteration in immune status) in addition to apparent transmission might be necessary for Hodgkin's disease to occur. In contrast to this study, Smith *et al.* (1974) examined the causes of death amongst 34 445 male doctors over a fifteen-year period in England and Wales and found no excess in this group. Additional studies will be required to resolve this matter.

Familial studies represent yet another indirect method of evaluating the transmission hypothesis. One of the first extensive investigations of familial Hodgkin's disease was conducted by Razis *et al.* (1959), who reviewed case records at Memorial Hospital, New York, between 1918 and 1958. Using cases of leukaemia, lymphosarcoma and other disorders as controls, they found a threefold excess of Hodgkin's disease among families with a member with this disorder. This was interpreted as being consistent with an infectious aetiology. Further evaluation (MacMahon, 1966) of this and another systematic study (DeVore and Doan, 1957) indicated that the two major familial patterns were sib–sib and parent–child and that most of these cases were under 40 years of age at diagnosis. MacMahon (1966) also suggested that if Hodgkin's disease is primarily a genetic disorder and has a definite age association, than the age of onset among sibs should be similar. Conversely, if environmental factors, particularly an infectious agent, are more important then the time interval between onsets of illness might reasonably be expected to be shorter than the age interval. Using the two major systematic familial studies of Hodgkin's disease, MacMahon (1966) found a greater similarity in time of onset than age of onset for sib cases; the mean time interval was 2·6 years whereas the mean difference between ages was 7·9 years. Since these familial studies were based on patient recall and records from single hospitals, the possibility exists that the familial cases identified might have been primarily those who were diagnosed close in time. To overcome this potential bias, an effort was made to identify instances of familial Hodgkin's disease among cases who lived in the same county ánd were reported to the tumour registry between 1950 and 1970 by using mortality and incidence data obtained from reports to the Cancer Control Bureau, New York State Department of Health (Vianna *et al.*, 1974c). Another potential source of familial cases employed was previously conducted surveys of all hospitals in four upstate New York counties. Twenty-three familial pairs (forty-six cases) were identified (Table 2.11) and used to evaluate the time and age intervals between diagnoses for first degree blood relatives and to test the hypothesis that the time interval between diagnoses for patients living in the same household might be shorter than that for patients of a similar relationship but living apart.

The age of patients ranged from 14 to 82 years, with thirty-one less than 40 years of age. Among the twenty-three familial cases diagnosed first there were sixteen males to seven females whereas the sex ratio was 13:10 for those diagnosed second. There were nine sib pairs, including one pair of identical twins, seven parent–child pairs and four instances where cases were related as cousins. The three remaining familial pairs were nephew–uncle, newphew–aunt and grandfather–grandaughter. No husband–wife pairs were observed. While there was no prevalent pattern of concordance or discordance by sex, only four couples were both female.

For seven of the nine sib pairs, the diagnostic time interval was significantly shorter than the difference between the ages at diagnosis. The median age interval was six years (mean 4·6 years, range 1–8 years) and the median interval between diagnosis was three years (mean 2·3 years, range 0·2–4 years). Parent–child pairs were obviously a generation apart in age but their median diagnostic interval was two years (mean 3·6 years, range 0·2–8·7 years).

Four parent–child and three sib pairs lived in the same household prior to and at the time the first case was diagnosed (group A). Of the sixteen familial pairs who resided in the same county but not the same household, nine (six sibs and three parent–child) were first degree relatives (group B). The median age of all group A cases was 31 years and for group B, 29 years. The median time interval between diagnoses

4—LM • •

Table 2.11 Age–sex, relationship, clinical site, Rye histological subtype, residential proximity and time interval between diagnoses of patients with familial Hodgkin's disease

| Couple no. | Source* | Case first diagnosed | | | Second case diagnosed | | | | Time interval between diagnoses (years) | Residence of second case before and after diagnosis of the first |
		Age at diagnosis and sex	Initial site	Rye subtype†	Relationship between cases	Age at diagnosis and sex	Initial site	Rye subtype†		
1	R	43M	cervical	MC	son–father	65M	axillary	MC	0·3	
2	R	20M	cervical	LD	brother–sister	18F	cervical	NS	3·0	
3	R	31M	spleen	LD	identical twin	32M	inguinal	LD	0·2	Group A
4	R	40F	cervical	—	mother–son	21M	cervical	—	0·0	same household
5	S	53M	cervical	—	father–son	23M	femoral	LP	1·0	
6	R	24M	cervical	LD	brothers	28M	axillary	LD	2·0	
7	R	18F	cervical	—	daughter–father	45M	cervical	—	2·0	
8	R	18M	cervical	—	son–father	50M	cervical	LD	8·6	
9	R	18M	submental	—	brothers	26M	cervical	LP/MC	3·0	
10	R	54M	cervical	LD	brothers	53M	supraclavicular	LD	4·0	
11	S	23M	cervical and inguinal	NS	brother–sister	29F	supraclavicular	NS	0·8	
12	R	41F	inguinal	NS	mother–daughter	16F	inguinal	MC	6·0	
13	R	41F	axillary	NS	mother–son	28M	cervical	NS	7·0	
14	S	35M	spleen	MC	brother–sister	29F	mediastinum	LD	3·3	
15	S	20F	cervical	LD	sisters	27F	supraclavicular	NS	3·3	Group B
16	S	80F	retroperitoneal	—	sisters	82F	cervical	LP/MC	1·0	same county
17	S	16M	cervical	MC	second cousins	31F	Supraclavicular	MC	5·0	
18	S	22F	supraclavicular	MC	distant cousins	22F	axillary	MC	4·7	
19	R	26M	mediastinal and cervical	NS/MC	distant cousins	33F	mediastinal and cervical	NS/MC	1·7	
20	S	29M	supraclavicular	LP	nephew–aunt	52F	supraclavicular	MC	1·0	
21	R	43M	cervical	—	uncle–nephew	24M	cervical	—	16·0	
22	R	23M	cervical	—	second cousins	43M	cervical	—	4·0	
23	S	72M	cervical	MC/LD	grandfather–granddaughter	14F	supraclavicular	NS	14·0	

* R = Registry, S = Survey
† MC = Mixed cellularity, LD = Lymphocyte depletion, LP = Lymphocyte predominance, NS = Nodular sclerosis, LP = Lymphocyte predominance (initial subtypes)

(From Vianna, N. J., Davies, J. N. P., Polan, A. et al, by courtesy of Lancet, 1974) for group A pairs was one year (mean 1·2 years, range 0·2–2 years) whereas for group B pairs it was 3·4 years (mean 4·1 years, range 0·8–8·7 years). The difference between the two groups was found to be statistically significant. A shorter diagnostic interval for group A cases was also apparent when sibs and parent–child pairs from each group were compared separately. These results should obviously be interpreted with caution since the number of familial cases identified was small. However, both studies that employed this approach (MacMahon, 1966; Vianna *et al.*, 1974b) have produced results that are compatible with the hypotheses that environmental factors are important in Hodgkin's disease. The possibility that the time interval between diagnoses for first degree blood related relatives might depend on their proximity to one another and not the specific nature of their relationship (e.g. sib–sib or parent–child) strongly favours an environmental and possibly infectious interpretation. Additional observations made in this study were that all four Rye subtypes were present among the fifteen familial pairs (Group A4, Group B11) in which the initial biopsy slides for both members were available (Table 2.11) and many of these pairs had concordant subtypes regardless of their relationship or proximity. This suggests that genetic factors might influence host reactivity, a possibility that gains support from the reported association between certain HL–A antigens and specific Rye subtypes (Falk and Osoba, 1971).

Taking a broad view of Hodgkin's disease, we are left with several considerations. Environmental factors are undoubtedly of major importance for all age groups with this disorder. There is a great deal of evidence which indicates a heterogeneity within this disease, especially between the childhood and adult age groups. The reasons behind these differences are unknown, but they must be viewed as dynamic, not fixed environmental factors. This seems clear since urbanisation with all its associated ramifications appears to underline and in many instances merge these differences together. Several hypotheses have been advanced which suggest that some form of transmission may be important in adult (young and old) Hodgkin's disease. These propositions all require further intensive evaluation and it must be realised that there is no easy way of doing this. Regardless of the approach taken, specific information will be required about each patient studied. Tumour registry data and hospital records, while important initial sources, are insufficient for this purpose. Patients must be interviewed. Available evidence also suggests the importance of host factors, environmental and genetic, in this disorder. Clearly not everyone who comes in contact with a patient develops Hodgkin's disease. If we constantly seek to determine how patients differ from others before they become ill, we will undoubtedly arrive at the cause(s) of Hodgkin's disease.

References

Alderson, M. R. and Nayak, R.: Epidemiology of Hodgkin's disease. *J. Chronic Dis.*, **25**:253, 1972.

Amiel, J. L.: Study of leukocyte phenotypes in Hodgkin's disease. In: *Histocompatibility Testing*, 79 (Copenhagen; Munksgaard: Baltimore, Williams and Wilkins, 1967).

Anderson, A. P., Brickner, H. and Lass, F.: Prognosis in Hodgkin's disease with special reference to histologic type. *Acta Radiol.*, **9**:81, 1970a.

Anderson, R. E., Ishida, K., Li, Y., Ishimaru, T. and Nishiyama, H.: Geographic aspects of malignant lymphoma and multiple myeloma. *Amer. J. Pathol.*, **61**:85, 1970b.

Bailar, J. C. and Gurian, J. M.: Month of birth and cancer mortality. *J. Nat. Cancer Inst.*, **33**:237, 1964.

Berard, C. W., Thomas, L. B., Axtell, L. M., Kruse, M., Newell, G. and Kagan, R.: The relationship of histopathologic subtype to clinical stage of Hodgkin's disease. *Cancer Res.*, **31**:1776, 1971.

Bjelke, E.: Hodgkin's disease in Norway. *Acta Med. Scand.*, **185**:73, 1969.

Bodmer, W. F.: Genetic factors in Hodgkin's disease: association with a disease susceptibility locus (DSA) in the HL-A region. In: *International Symposium on Hodgkin's Disease*, 36 (Washington, D.C.: U.S. Government Printing Office, 1972, 127) (National Cancer Institute Monograph).

Braylan, R., Pascuccelli, H., Stadecker, M. and Morgenfeld, M. C.: Hodgkin's disease—a report from Buenos Aires, Argentina. *Cancer*, **32**:879, 1973.

Brit. Med. J., editorial: Hodgkin's disease: a clue or a fluke? **4**:564, 1972.

Bross, I. D. J., Shimaoka, K. and Tidings, J.: Some epidemiologic clues in thyroid cancer: tonsillectomy, acne, allergy and ethnicity. *Arch. Int. Med.*, **128**:755, 1971.

Burn, C., Davies, J. N. P., Dodge, O. G. and Nias, B. C.: Hodgkin's disease in English and African children. *J. Nat. Cancer Inst.*, **46**:37, 1971.

Chang, A.: Enfermedad de Hodgkin: histopathologia. *Acta Cancerologica*, (*Lima*), **6**:30, 1967.

Chism, S. E., Order, S. E. and Hellman, S.: Tumor-fetal antigens in Hodgkin's disease: an immunoelectrophoretic analysis. *Amer. J. Roentgenol. Radium Therm. Nucl. Med.*, **117**:51, 1973.

Cole, P., MacMahon, B. and Aisenberg, A.: Mortality from Hodgkin's disease in the United States. *Lancet*, **2**:1371, 1968.

Cole, P., Mack, T., Rothman, K. *et al.*: Tonsillectomy and Hodgkin's disease. *New Eng. J. Med.*, **288**:634, 1973.

Correa, P.: *International Symposium on Hodgkin's Disease*, 36 (Washington, D.C.: U.S. Government Printing Office, 1972, 9) (National Cancer Institute Monograph).

Correa, P. and O'Conor, G. T.: Epidemiologic patterns of Hodgkin's disease. *Int. J. Cancer*, **8**:192, 1971.

Cridland, M. D.: Seasonal incidence of clinical onset of Hodgkin's disease. *Brit. Med. J.*, **2**:621, 1961.

Davies, J. N. P. and Owor, R.: Chloromatous tumors in African children in Uganda. *Brit. Med. J.*, **2**:405, 1965.

DeVore, J. W. and Doan, C. A.: A study of the Hodgkin's syndrome XII. Hereditary and epidemiological aspects. *Ann. Int. Med.*, **47**:300, 1957.

DiPietro, S. and Pizzetti, F.: La prognosi istoloica del granuloma maligno in base allo studio di 100 casi. *Tumori*, **52**:451, 1966.

Doll, R., Muir, C. and Waterhouse, J. (editors): *Cancer in Five Continents, 2,* (New York: Springer-Verlag, 1970).

Dorfman, R. F.: Relationship of histology to site in Hodgkin's disease. *Cancer Res.*, **31**:1786, 1971.

Dörken, H. and Singer-Bakker, H.: Hodgkin's disease in childhood—an edpidemiologic study in Northern Germany. In: *Current Problems in the Epidemiology of Cancer and Lymphomas*, 1st Ed., 235 (E. Grundmann and H. Tullinius, editors) (Berlin, Heidelberg, New York, Springer-Verlag, 1972).

Dworsky, R. L. and Henderson, B. E.: Hodgkin's disease clustering in families and communities. *Cancer Res.*, **34**:1161, 1974.

Falk, J. and Osoba, D.: HL-A antigens and survival in Hodgkin's disease. *Lancet*, **2**:1118, 1971.

Fasal, E., Jackson, E. W. and Klauber, M. R.: Leukemia and lymphoma mortality and farm residence. *Amer. J. Epidemiol.*, **87**:267, 1968.

Forbes, J. F. and Morris, P. J.: Leukocyte antigens in Hodgkin's disease. *Lancet*, **2**:849, 1970.

Forbes, J. F. and Morris, P. J.: Analysis of HL-A antigens in patients with Hodgkin's disease and their families. *J. Clin. Invest.*, **51**:1156, 1972.

Franssila, K. O., Kalima, T. V. and Voutilainen, A.: Histologic classifications of Hodgkin's disease. *Cancer*, **20**: 1594, 1967.

Fraumeni, J. F. and Li, F. P.: Hodgkin's disease in childhood; an epidemiologic study. *J. Nat. Cancer Inst.*, **42**:681, 1969.

Gough, J.: Hodgkin's disease; a correlation of histopathology with survival. *Int. J. Cancer*, **5**:273, 1970.

Hamann, W., Oehlert, W., Musshoff, K., Nuss, A. and Schnellbacher, B.: The histologic classification of Hodgkin's disease and its relevance to prognosis. *Germ. Med. Mon.*, **15**:509, 1970.

Hanson, T. A. S.: Histologic classification and survival in Hodgkin's disease. *Cancer*, **17**:1595, 1964.

Hartwich, G. and Schlabeck, H.: Lymphogranulomatose: Jahreszeitliche verteilung der erstmanifestation. *Dtsch. Med. Wochenschr.*, **95**:1387, 1970.

Hodgkin, T.: On some morbid appearances of the absorbent glands and spleen. *Med. Chir. Trans.*, **17**:68, 1832.

Innes, J. and Newall, J.: Seasonal incidence in clinical onset of Hodgkin's disease. *Brit. Med. J.*, **2**:765, 1961.

Jelliffe, A. M. and Thompson, A. D.: The prognosis in Hodgkin's disease. *Brit. J. Cancer*, **9**:21, 1955.

Johnson, S. K. and Johnson, R. E.: Tonsillectomy history in Hodgkin's disease. *New Eng. J. Med.*, **287**:1122, 1972.

Kissmeyer-Nielsen, F., Jensen, K. B. and Ferrara, G. B.: HL-A phenotypes in Hodgkin's disease: preliminary report. *Transpl. Proc.*, **3**:1287, 1971.

Klinger, R. J. and Minton, J. P.: Case clustering of Hodgkin's disease in a small rural community with associations among cases. *Lancet*, **1**:168, 1973.

Landberg, T. and Larsson, L.: Hodgkin's disease. *Acta Radiol.*, **8**:390, 1969.

Lukes, R. J., Butler, J. J. and Hicks, E. B.: Natural history of Hodgkin's disease as related to its pathologic picture. *Cancer*, **19**:317, 1966.

Mallory, F. B.: *Principles of Pathologic Histology*, **2** (Philadelphia: W. B. Saunders, 1914).

MacMahon, B.: Epidemiology of Hodgkin's disease. *Cancer Res.*, **26**:1189, 1966.

Meytes, D. and Modan, B.: Selected aspects of Hodgkin's disease in a whole community. *Blood*, **34**:91, 1969.

Milham, S.: Hodgkin's disease in teachers. *New Eng. J. Med.*, **290**:1329, 1974.

Miller, R. W.: Mortality in childhood Hodgkin's disease. An etiologic clue. *J.A.M.A.*, **198**:216, 1966.

Neiman, R. S., Rosen, P. J. and Lukes, R. J.: Lymphocyte-depletion Hodgkin's disease: a clinicopathological entity. *New Eng. J. Med.*, **288**:751, 1973.

Newall, J.: The management of Hodgkin's disease. *Clin. Radiol.*, **16**:40, 1965.

Newall, G. R.: Seasonal onset of Hodgkin's disease. *Lancet*, **1**:1024, 1972.

Newall, G. R., Rawlings, W., Kinnear, B. K. *et al.*: Case–control study of Hodgkin's disease. 1. Results of the interview questionnaire. *J. Nat. Cancer Inst.*, **51**:1437, 1973.

Nickels, J., Franssila, K. and Hjelt, L.: Thymoma and Hodgkin's disease of the thymus. *Acta Pathol. et Microbiol. Scand. A.*, **81**:1, 1973.

O'Conor, G. T., Correa, P., Christine, B., Axtell, L. and Myers, M.: *International Symposium on Hodgkin's Disease*, 36 (Washington, D.C.: U.S. Government Printing Office, 1972, 3) (National Cancer Institute Monograph).

Olweny, C. L. M., Ziegler, J. L., Berard, C. W. *et al.*: Adult Hodgkin's disease in Uganda. *Cancer*, **27**:1295, 1971.

Order, S. E., Chism, S. E. and Hellman, S.: Studies of antigens associated with Hodgkin's disease. *Blood*, **40**:621, 1972.

Pike, M. C., Henderson, B. E., Casagrande, J., Smith, P. G. and Kinlen, L. J.: Infectious aspects of Hodgkin's disease. *New Eng. J. Med.*, **290**:341, 1974.

Pike, M. C. and Smith, P. G.: Tonsillectomy and Hodgkin's disease. *Lancet*, **1**:434, 1973.

Piperno, J. R. and Kallen, R. G.: Evidence for multiple forms of DNA polymerase in Hodgkin's disease. *Cancer Res.*, **33**:838, 1973.

Rappaport, H., Strum, S. B., Hutchinson, G. and Allen, L. W.: Clinical and biologic significance of vascular invasion in Hodgkin's disease. *Cancer Res.*, **31**:1794, 1971.

Razis, D. V., Diamond, H. D. and Craver, L. F.: Familial Hodgkin's disease: its significance and implications. *Ann. Int. Med.*, **51**:933, 1959.

Reed, D. M.: On the pathological changes in Hodgkin's disease with especial reference to its relation to tuberculosis. *Johns Hopkins Hosp. Rep.*, **10**:133, 1902.

Ruuskanen, O., Vanha-Pertulla, T. and Kouvalainen, K.: Tonsillectomy, appendectomy and Hodkgin's disease. *Lancet*, **1**:1127, 1971.

Selzer, G., Kahn, L. B. and Sealy, R.: Hodgkin's disease, a clinicopathologic study of 122 cases. *Cancer*, **29**:1090, 1972.

Shimaoka, K., Bross, I. D. J. and Tidings, J.: Tonsillectomy and Hodgkin's disease. *New Eng. J. Med.*, **288**:634, 1973.

Shimkin, M. B.: Mortality in the United States, 1921–1951; race, sex, and age distribution; comparison with leukemia. *Blood*, **10**:1214, 1955.

Smith, P. G., Kinle, L. J. and Doll, R.: Hodgkin's disease mortality among physicians. *Lancet*, **2**:525, 1974.

Smithers, D. W.: Hodgkin's disease: one entity or two? *Lancet*, **2**:1285, 1970.

Smither's, D. W.: Summary of informal discussion of biostatistical and epidemiologic factors in Hodgkin's disease. *Cancer Res.*, **31**:1866, 1971.

Solidoro, A., Guzman, C. and Chang, A.: Relative increased incidence of childhood Hodgkin's disease in Peru. *Cancer Res.*, **26**:1204, 1966.

Stalsberg, H.: Hodgkin's disease in Western Europe: a review. In: *International Symposium of Hodgkin's Disease*, 36 (Washington, D.C.: U.S. Government Printing Office, 1972, 31) (National Cancer Institute Monograph).

Sternberg, C.: Uber line ligenartige unter dem Bilde der pseudoleukamie verlaufende tuberculose des lymphatischen apparates. *Ztschr. Heilk.*, **19**:21, 1898.

Strum, S. B. and Rappaport, H.: Interrelations of the histologic types of Hodgkin's disease. *Arch. Pathol.*, **91**:127. 1971a.

Strum, S. B. and Rappaport, H.: The persistence of Hodgkin's disease in long-term survivors. *Amer. J. Med.*, **51**:222, 1971b.

The Registrar-General's Decennial Supplement, England and Wales, 1961. Occupational mortality tables, 418 (London: H.M.S.O., 1971).

Thomas, L. B. and Berard, C. W.: Relationship of histopathologic type at diagnosis to clinical parameters and to histologic distribution at autopsy. *GANN*, **15**:253, 1973.

Uhl, N. Hauswaldt, C. and Hungstein, W.: Jahreszeitliche Verteilung der erstmanifestation der lymphogranulomatose. *Verh. Dtsch. Ges. Inn. Med.*, **73**:329, 1967.

Vianna, N. J., Davies, J. N. P., Polan, A. and Wolfgang, P.: Hodgkin's disease: an environmental and genetic disorder. *Lancet*, 1974c **2**:854, 1974.

Vianna. N. J., Greenwald, P., Brady, J., Polan, A. K. *et al.*: Hodgkin's disease: cases with features of a community outbreak. *Ann. Int. Med.*, **77**:169, 1972.

Vianna, N. J., Greenwald, P. and Davies, J. N. P.: Tonsillectomy and Hodgkin's disease: the lymphoid tissue barrier. *Lancet*, **1**:431, 1971a.

Vianna, N. J., Greenwald, P. and Davies, J. N. P.: Extended epidemic of Hodgkin's disease in high school students. *Lancet*, **1**:1209, 1971b.

Vianna, N. J., Greenwald, P., Polan, A. *et al.*: Tonsillectomy and Hodgkin's disease. *Lancet*, **2**:168, 1974a.

Vianna, N. J. and Polan, A. K.: Epidemiologic evidence for transmission of Hodgkin's disease. *New Eng. J. Med.*, **289**:499, 1973.

Vianna, N. J., Polan, A. K., Keogh, M. D. and Greenwald, P.: Hodgkin's disease mortality among physicians. *Lancet*, **2**:131, 1974b.

Wakasa, H.: Hodgkin's disease in Asia, particularly in Japan. *Internatonal Symposium on Hodgkin's Disease*, 36 (Washington, D.C.: U.S. Government Printing Office, 1972, 15) (National Cancer Institute Monograph).

Warthin, A. S.: Genetic neoplastic relationships of Hodgkin's disease, aleukemic and leukemic lymphoblastoma, and mycosis fungoides. *Ann. Surg.*, **93**:153, 1931.

Wilks, Sir S.: Cases of enlargement of the lymphatic glands and spleen (or, Hodgkin's disease), with remarks. *Guy's Hosp. Rep.*, **11**:56, 1865.

Wright, D. H.: Epidemiology and histology of Hodgkin's disease in Uganda. *International Symposium on Hodgkin's Disease*, 36 (Washington, D.C.: U.S. Government Printing Office, 1972, 23) (National Cancer Institute Monograph).

Zervas, J. D., Delamore, J. W. and Israels, M. C.: Leucocyte phenotypes in Hodgkin's disease. *Lancet*, **2**:634, 1970.

CHAPTER 3

Burkitt's lymphoma

Burkitt's lymphoma is one of the few lymphoreticular malignancies for which specific aetiologic hypotheses have been proposed. Furthermore there is general agreement that this tumour has certain cytologic and histologic features which distinguish it from the other lymphomas (Berard *et al.*, 1969). It is the most frequently encountered childhood malignancy in tropical Africa and has an endemic pattern in countries such as Uganda (Burkitt and Davies, 1961) and New Guinea (Booth *et al.*, 1967). This contrasts with the sporadic occurrence of this disorder in Canada, Great Britain, the United States and Brazil (Hoogstraten, 1965; Dorfman, 1965; Wright, 1966; Besuschio, 1974). In addition to these marked international variations in incidence, other differences have been observed. Cases reported in the United States have a median age of about 10 years (Cohen *et al.*, 1969) and a relatively broad age range. In countries with an endemic pattern, the mean age is 8 years and the age range is considerably smaller (Burkitt and O'Conor, 1967). Interestingly, the age distribution among Africans from non-endemic areas closely approximates that found in America. In areas where this tumour occurs sporadically, there is a low incidence of jaw tumours and abdominal tumours dominate the clinical picture. Peripheral lymphadenopathy has been observed in approximately 30 per cent of American cases (Cohen *et al.*, 1969). In endemic areas the majority of cases have maxillary or mandibular tumours at onset and peripheral lymphadenopathy is rarely present (Burkitt and O'Conor, 1961). These contrasting patterns are most intriguing in view of the histologic similarity of Burkitt's tumour in endemic and non-endemic areas (Cohen *et al.*, 1969).

Several additional features of this tumour are indicative of its unique character. Haddow (1963) showed that in Africa Burkitt's lymphoma occurred with the greatest frequency in regions with a mean temperature of 60 °F or greater during the coolest month, and an average rainfall of not less than 20 inches a year. New Guinea has similar climatic features.

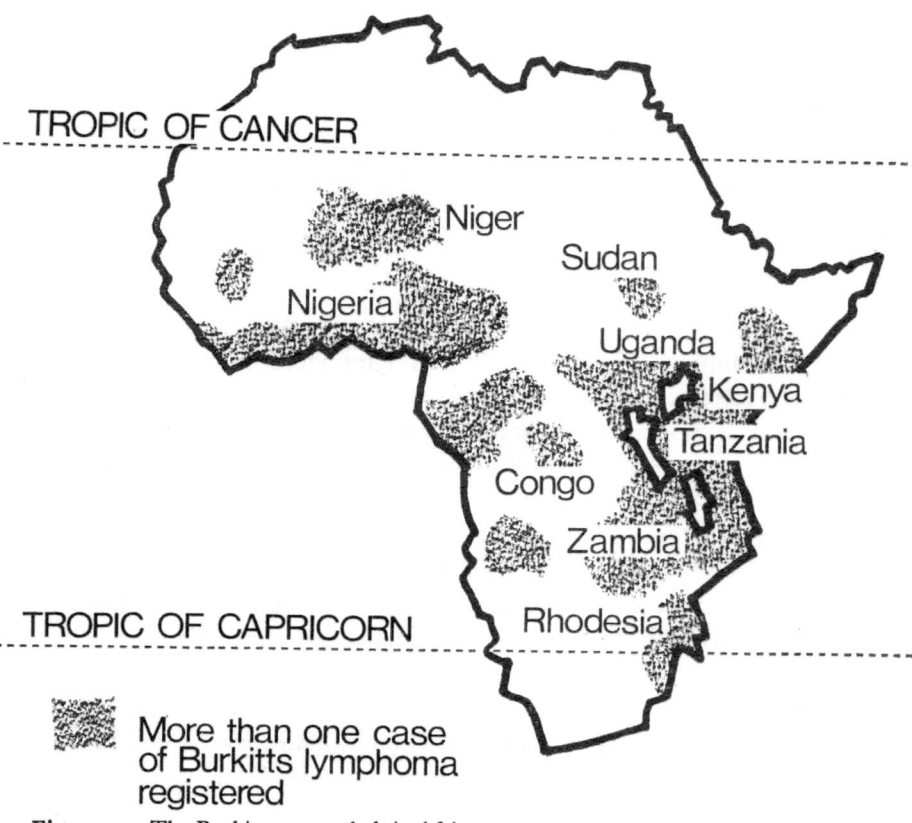

Figure 3.1 The Burkitt tumour belt in Africa

However on the Ivory Coast where this disease is endemic in sylvanic zones and rare in the prairies, no significant differences were observed in rainfall or median or maximum temperatures (Loubiere, 1974). In both regions, however, marked differences in the curves of minimal temperature and relative humidity were found. Other observations suggest that the disease occurs frequently around lakes but not in mountain regions with altitudes above 5000 feet (Burkitt and Davies, 1961). None of the other lymphomas show the climatic dependence of the Burkitt tumour. Even within the Burkitt tumour belt in Africa (Figure 3.1), the incidence of this disorder is quite variable (Burkitt, 1967). Another important point is that this is not a tumour of African children but rather one of children in Africa; neither racial nor tribal characteristics appear to affect tumour incidence (Burkitt, 1963).

TIME–SPACE CLUSTERING

Significant time–space clustering has been demonstrated in the West Nile district and Bwamba (Pike *et al.*, 1967). Additional evidence was presented that the occurrence of case clusters during certain years moved from county to county. This phenomenon of epidemic drift suggested that some environmental agent moved through the community. A more recent study failed to find evidence of clustering in the North Mara district of Tanzania, a high risk area (Brubaker *et al.*, 1973). Additional studies will be required to further evaluate the possibility that clustering occurs in this disorder but unfortunately the rarity with which it occurs makes it impossible to conduct this type of investigation in areas other than Africa and New Guinea. One possible explanation for the discrepancy in results might be that clustering of cases does not occur in this disorder. It is equally possible that inappropriate time or place co-ordinates were employed in both instances. Before additional studies are initiated, it might be worth while to consider a few underlying questions. Since this is primarily a childhood disorder, the induction period might be relatively small. Is there any evidence to suggest seasonality either by month of birth or onset? Williams *et al.* (1974) examined the possibility that a seasonal variation in month of onset of Burkitt's lymphoma might exist in the West Nile district of Uganda. Their results suggested that about 80 per cent more cases occurred in the second half of the year than in the first half. However, examination of the onset of cases by single month indicates that during July, November and many months of the first half of the year, a similar number of cases occurred. Furthermore, while seasonality was clearly apparent in the north–south direction, it was not apparent in the east–west division of the area studied. The impact that these preliminary observations might have on future time–space cluster studies seems obvious. Further evaluation of a possible seasonal influence in Burkitt's lymphoma is essential and should be given a high priority. The high frequency of this tumour in parts of tropical Africa can be taken as evidence of space clustering but it clearly does not localise the specific place co-ordinate. Could it be place of birth? Another important consideration relates to possible contact patterns of cases. Can patients with this disorder be associated with one another? The only available approach to this question at the present time is to evaluate clusters of Burkitt's lymphoma. Evaluation of the African clusters (Pike *et al.*, 1967·

Williams *et al.*, 1969; Morrow *et al.*, 1971), all of which occurred in Uganda, reveals little evidence to suggest case–to–case horizontal transmission. In the Bwamba County cluster, however, which consisted of seven cases diagnosed over a twenty-seven-month period, two patients were brother and sister, aged 9 and 3 years respectively (Morrow *et al.*, 1971). Of interest is the fact that the interval between onsets of illness for these sibs was about six months. Although another report refers to two sisters in Kenya, their ages and dates of onset were not specified (Daldorf *et al.*, 1964). In the United States there have been few reported groupings of Burkitt lymphoma cases. One cluster involved two boys, 9 and 15 years of age and both presented with pharyngeal tumours during the same month and year (Levine *et al.*, 1973). Remarkably, although they lived only three houses apart, the boys were not acquainted. Another reported group involved a pair of sibs from southern California, who developed Burkitt's tumour simultaneously (Stevens *et al.*, 1972). The sister in this group was 17 years old at onset and her brother was 8 years of age. Thus, the age interval between onsets was greater than the time interval, as was true for the African sibs with this disorder. While both observations are more consistent with an environmental rather than a genetic–age associated disorder, more familial cases will be required to evaluate time and age intervals between onsets. This approach would yield valuable information about the relative importance of genetic and environmental factors in Burkitt's lymphoma; it might also provide us with important clues as to the specific time and place of exposure. Although evaluation of the few reported clusters of Burkitt's lymphoma in Africa and the United States might be interpreted as being inconsistent with case–case transmission, the possibility of horizontal and/or vertical transmission in humans requires more intensive study. Admittedly this concept is difficult to evaluate epidemiologically but it is fundamental to our understanding the pathogenesis of this disorder. If for example Burkitt's lymphoma is a mosquito-borne disorder, one might observe clustering, an endemic pattern in certain areas but not others, and epidemic drift but no significant associations among cases. Where human transmission is important be it direct (case–case) or indirect through some healthy carrier (case–intermediary–case or maternal–fetal infection–childhood case), cases should be related in some manner. Furthermore, if the induction period is long and/or significant migration occurs, time–space clustering, endemic patterns and epidemic drift might not be expected.

AETIOLOGIC CONSIDERATIONS

Both the geographic localisation and climatic dependence of the Burkitt tumour suggested that some vector–borne viral agent might play a causal role (Haddow, 1963; Burkitt and Wright, 1966). This led to an intensive search for a virus in tumour tissue. Although several viral agents, including Rheo 3 (Bell *et al.*, 1966) and herpes simplex (Simons and Ross, 1965), were either isolated or considered, the Epstein–Barr virus (EBV) emerged as the most likely candidate on the basis of sero-epidemiologic evidence (Epstein and Barr, 1965). However, it became apparent that EBV is worldwide in distribution, including remote tribes in Brazil (Evans and Niderman, 1971) and Alaska (Tischendorf *et al.*, 1970). Studies in several countries have further indicated that the prevalence of EBV antibody varies according to the level of socio-economic development. Another important concept is that the occurrence of clinical infectious mononucleosis in a country is inversely related to the age at which infection occurs (Evans and Niederman, 1971). Thus, clinical infectious mononucleosis is a disorder of developed countries such as the United States, Great Britain and Canada but not South American or African countries, where EBV is more prevalent at an earlier age (Evans and Niederman, 1971). But whereas EBV infection is widespread, the Burkitt tumour is not. This suggested that EBV infection alone could not be the cause of the Burkitt tumour; additional factor(s) had to be involved. In recent years evidence has been presented to suggest that malaria might be an important co-factor. Daldorf *et al.* (1964) were the first to suggest this possible relationship and this hypothesis gained support by the observation that in Uganda there was a close association between the incidence of Burkitt's lymphoma and malariometric indices (Burkitt, 1969; O'Conor, 1970). It has also been suggested that the incidence of this tumour has declined in those areas where malaria control has been instituted (Baikie *et al.*, 1972). Furthermore, although there are proven exceptions, it is generally agreed that malaria gametocytes cannot develop successfully within the body of the mosquito host when the average temperature is below 60 °F, (Herms and James, 1961) an observation which fits well with climatic factors described for this tumour. However, it is extremely difficult to explain a rare event such as the Burkitt tumour by invoking yet an additional common event such as malaria infection. It is also possible that malaria control might have resulted in the simultaneous eradication of some other vector-borne viral agent. Another difficulty with the EBV-malaria hypothesis becomes obvious when one finds occasional cases of this disorder in countries, such as the United States, where malaria rarely occurs. Furthermore, there may be no significant difference in EBV titres between American Burkitt lymphoma cases and controls and one-third of these cases have no EBV antibody titre (Hirshaut *et al.*, 1973). To confound matters further, an increase in EBV titre has been reported in patients with other diseases. In the lymphocyte depleted stage of Hodgkin's disease (Levine *et al.*, 1971), nasopharyngeal carcinoma (Henle *et al.*, 1970), and even sarcoidosis (Hirchaut *et al.*, 1970) antibody levels are comparable to those found in Burkitt's lymphoma. Thus, despite rather strong circumstantial evidence, the possibility that EBV might be only a passenger virus in Burkitt's lymphoma must also be considered.

What can be made of these apparently conflicting observations? Invoking additional co-factors seems useless since we can not explain the two factors already identified. It is possible that Burkitt's lymphoma is a single entity in both Africa and Western countries but that it is caused by some totally unknown factor(s). It is equally possible that EBV and malaria are aetiologically associated with this tumour in African countries but not in the United States. This concept of a dual aetiology gains some support from the differences in this disorder observed in countries with endemic and non-endemic patterns. But the evidence implicating EBV and Burkitt's tumour, while admittedly circumstantial, is strong. EBV–DNA has been found in cultured tumour cells (Zur-Hausen, 1970) and hybridisation experiments indicate that all Burkitt cells contain the EBV genome (Zur-Hausen and Schulte-Holthausen, 1970). Perhaps the difficulties encountered with the EBV-Burkitt tumour hypothesis revolve around our poor understanding of the effects of EBV infection, especially in the immunologically incompetent host. Another important consideration might be the time of exposure. Susceptibility to many viruses varies with age and this also holds true for EBV. This virus causes infectious mononucleosis in adolescents and young adults (Niederman, 1956) but asymptomatic infection in both these and childhood age groups (Sutton *et al.*, 1974). Little is known of the effects of chronic infection with EBV in these individuals. Even less is known about the effects of fetal infection with this virus. Considering that the Burkitt lymphoma is predominantly a childhood disorder, the possibility that exposure during this period might be important, should be considered. Social factors are also of obvious importance for they influence the age pattern of EBV infection. How does the socio-economic status of cases in endemic and non-endemic areas compare? If EBV is associated with Burkitt's lymphoma, the answer to this question might provide some clue as to the important time of exposure to this agent.

What then can be said about malaria as a co-factor? If another factor is indeed required, it seems clear that environmental factors other than malaria must be sought, at least in countries such as the United States and Great Britain. Since partial immunosuppression by malaria has been demonstrated experimentally and in man, other agents capable of the same action in Western countries must be sought.

RELATIONSHIP BETWEEN BURKITT'S TUMOUR AND ACUTE LYMPHATIC LEUKAEMIA

It is perhaps premature to consider the possible association between Burkitt's lymphoma and other lymphocytic malignancies, but this has been the subject of much controversy and such an exercise might be useful to our understanding of certain of these disorders. The major issue centres around the hypothesis that acute lymphoblastic leukaemia and Burkitt's lymphoma are alternative forms of one another. The proponents of this hypothesis point out that lymphoblastic leukaemia is the major childhood lymphoproliferative malignancy in the northern hemisphere, whereas, in much of Africa and New Guinea Burkitt's lymphoma predominates (O'Conor and Davies, 1960; Stewart *et al.*, 1973). They further point out that in certain African countries there is a deficiency of acute lymphoblastic leukaemia (Templeton, 1973) and suggest that this deficiency might occur in those areas where Burkitt's lymphoma is most common. While some (Vanier and Pike, 1967) have argued that this apparent leukaemic deficiency is due to under-diagnosis or incomplete ascertainment, several recent studies have also found low rates for childhood lymphatic leukaemia in various parts of Africa. In Mulago Hospital, Templeton (1973) found a deficiency of this subtype but not the other varieties of acute leukaemia. In Rhodesia, Lowe (1974) found a similar deficit. Amsel and Nabembezi (1974) conducted a two-year survey of haematologic malignancies in Uganda and also found a low incidence of childhood lymphatic leukaemia (Figure 3.2). However, this study also showed that in areas such as Kyadondo county, the incidence of both this leukaemic subtype and Burkitt's lymphoma was low. It seems that a deficiency in childhood lymphatic leukaemia in

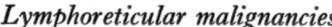

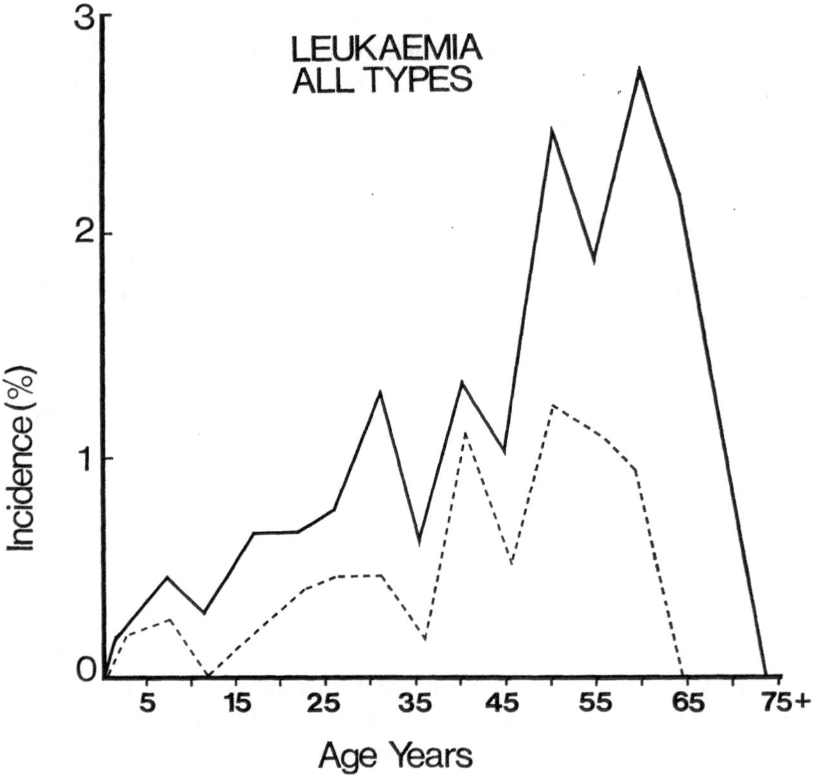

Figure 3.2 Age–specific incidence curve of leukaemia in Uganda, 1971 and 1972
——— Male, - - - - Female.

certain African countries does exist, but the incidence of this disorder is not inversely related to that of Burkitt's lymphoma. Of course these observations neither prove nor disprove a possible association between the two diseases. Perhaps the strongest argument against the unitarian hypothesis is that the age incidence of the two disorders differs, acute lymphoblastic leukaemia peaking around the third year and the Burkitt's tumour around the seventh year of life. There is need for further studies of the incidence of different subtypes of childhood leukaemia and Burkitt's lymphoma in various regions of Africa. If some relationship is demonstrated, this would provide evidence supporting the possibility that some exposure during gestation might be essential in the Burkitt tumour, for available evidence (Chapter 5) suggests that this might be the case with acute lymphatic leukaemia in childhood. Another dividend that might be gained from this type of study is the further evaluation of the possible role of environmental factors, such as malaria in Burkitt's lymphoma. Thus, a lymphatic leukaemia phase has been reported in Burkitt's lymphoma (Levine *et al.*, 1973) and interestingly this transition appears to be more common in American cases (Cohen *et al.*, 1969) than in African. Is malaria a localising factor in Africa? If so this might explain why Burkitt's lymphoma acts in somewhat of a similar fashion to lymphosarcoma in America (Dorfman, 1968). Interestingly these two lymphomas have certain histologic features in common, both have childhood incidence peaks at later ages than that for leukaemia and both have been reported to undergo leukaemia transition in America.

References

Amsel, S. and Nabembezi, J. S.: Two-year survey of hematologic malignancies in Uganda. *J. Nat. Cancer Inst.*, **52**:1397, 1974.

Baikie, A. G., Kinlen, L. J. and Pike, M. C.: Detection and assessment of case clustering in Burkitt's lymphoma and Hodgkin's disease. In: *Current Problems in the Epidemiology of Cancer and Lymphomas*, 201 (E. Grundmann, and H. Tullinius, editors) (Berlin, Heidelberg, New York,: Springer-Verlag, 1972).

Bell, T. M., Massie, A., Ross, M. G. R. *et al.*: Isolation of reovirus from a case of Burkitt's lymphoma. *Brit. Med. J.*, **1**:1514, 1966.

Berard, C. W., *et al.* editors: Histopathological definition of Burkitt's tumor. *Bull. WHO*, **40**:601, 1969.

Besuschio, S. C.: Geographic pathology of lymphomas in Latin America. *Medicina*, **34**:31, 1974.

Booth, K., Burkitt, D. P., Bassett, D. J., Cooke, R. A. *et al.*: Burkitt lymphoma in Papua New Guinea. *Brit. J. Cancer*, **21**:657, 1967.

Brubaker, G., Geser, A. and Pike, M.: Burkitt's lymphoma in the North Mara district of Tanzania, 1964–1970: failure to find evidence of time–space clustering in a high risk isolated rural area. *Brit. J. Cancer*, **28**:469, 1973.

Burkitt, D.: A lymphoma syndrome dependant on environment. In: *Symposium on Lymphoreticular Tumors in Africa*, 80 (F. C., Rowlet, editor) (Basel, New York, S. Karger, 1963).

Burkitt, D. P.: Recent developments in geographic distribution. In: *Treatment of Burkitt's tumor*, 33 (J. H. Burchenal, and D. P. Burkitt, editors) (Berlin, Heidelberg, New York: Springer-Verlag, 1967).

Burkitt, D. P.: Etiology of Burkitt's lymphoma—an alternative hypothesis to a vectoral virus. *J. Nat. Cancer Inst.*, **42**:19, 1969.

Burkitt, D. P. and Davies, J. N. P.: Lymphoma syndrome in Uganda and tropical Africa. *Afr. Med. Press*, **245**:367, 1961.

Burkitt, D. P. and O'Conor, G. T.: Malignant lymphoma in African children: I. Clinical syndrome. *Cancer*, **14**:258, 1961.

Burkitt, D. P. and O'Conor, G. T.: *UICC Symposium on the treatment of Burkitt's tumor*, 2 (New York: Springer-Verlag, 1967).

Burkitt, D. P. and Wright, D. H.: Geographic and tribal distribution of African lymphoma in Uganda. *Brit. Med. J.*, **1**:569, 1966.

Cohen, M. H., Bennett, J. M., Berard, C. W., Ziegler, J. L. *et al.*: Burkitt's tumor in the United States. *Cancer*, **23**:1259, 1969.

Daldorf, G., Linsell, C. A., Barnhart, F. E. *et al.*: An epidemiologic approach to the lymphomas of African children and Burkitt's sarcoma of the jaws. *Perspect. Biol. Med.* **7**:435, 1964.

Dorfman, R. F.: Childhood lymphosarcoma in St. Louis, Missouri, clinically and histologically resembling Burkitt's tumor. *Cancer*, **18**:418, 1965.

Dorfman, R. F.: Diagnosis of Burkitt's tumor in the United States. *Cancer*, **21**:563, 1968.

Epstein, M. A., Barr, Y. M., Achong, B. G.: Studies with Burkitt's lymphoma. *Wistar. Inst. Symp. Monog.* **4**:69, 1965.

Evans, A. S., Niederman, J. C.: Epidemiology of infectious mononucleosis. In: Proc. *Symposium in Oncogenesis and Herpes-type Viruses, Cambridge, England*, 1971 (June).

Haddow, A. J.: An improved map for the study of Burkitt's lymphoma syndrome in Africa. *East Afr. Med. J.*, **40**-429, 1963.

Henle, W., Henle, G., Ho, H. *et al.*: Antibodies to Epstein–Barr virus in nasopharyngeal carcinoma, other head and neck neoplasms and control groups. *J. Nat. Cancer Inst.* **44**:225, 1970.

Herms, W. B. and James, M. T.: Mosquitoes as vectors of disease. In: *Medical Entomology*, 195 (New York, Macmillan Company, 1961).

Hirshaut, Y., Cohen, M. H. and Stevens, D. A.: Epstein–Barr virus antibodies in American and African Burkitt's lymphoma. *Lancet*, **2**:114, 1973.

Hirshaut, Y., Glade, P., Vieria, L. O. *et al.*: Sarcoidosis, another disease associated with serologic evidence for herpes-like virus infection. *New Eng. J. Med.*, **283**:502, 1970.

Hoogstraten, J.: The occurrence of Burkitt's African childhood lymphosarcoma in central Canada. *J. Pediat.* **67**:1015, 1965.

Levine, P. H., Ablashi, D. V and Berard, C. W.: Elevated antibody titers to Epstein–Barr virus in Hodgkin's disease. *Cancer*, **27**:416, 1971.

Levine, P. H., Sandler, S. G., Komp, D. M. *et al.*: Simultaneous occurrence of American Burkitt's lymphoma in neighbors. *New Eng. J. Med.*, **288**:562, 1973.

Loubiere, R: Geographic pathology of Burkitt lymphoma on the Ivory Coast. *Medicina*, **34**:32, 1974.

Lowe, R. F.: Leukemia in Rhodesian Africa. *Cent. Afr. J. Med.*, **20**: 80, 1974.

Morrow, R. H., Pike, M. C., Smith, P. G. *et al.*: Burkitt's lymphoma: a time-space cluster of cases in Bwamba County of Uganda. *Brit. Med. J.*, **2**:491, 1971.

Niederman, J. C.: Infectious monocucleosis at Yale-New Haven Medical Center, 1946–1955. *Yale J. Biol. Med.*, **28**:629, 1956.

O'Conor, G. T.: Persistent immunologic stimulation as a factor in oncogenesis, with special reference to Burkitt's tumors. *Amer. J. Med.*, **48**:279, 1970.

O'Conor, G. T. and Davies, J. N. P.: Malignant tumors in African children: with special reference to malignant lymphoma. *J, Pediat.* **56**:526, 1960.

Pike, M. C., Williams, E. H. and Wright, D.: Burkitt's tumor in the West Nile District of Uganda 1961–1965. *Brit. Med. J.*, **2**:395, 1967.

Simons, P. J., and Ross, M. G. R.: Isolation of herpes virus from Burkitt's tumors. *Eur. J. Cancer*, **1**:135. 1965.

Stevens, D. A., O'Conor, G. T., Levine, P. H. *et al.*: Acute leukemia with Burkitt's lymphoma cells and Burkitt's lymphoma. *Ann. Int. Med.*, **76**:967, 1972.

Stewart, A., Davies, J. N. P., Dalldorf, G. *et al.*: Malignant lymphomas of African children. *Proc. Nat. Acad. Sci.*, **70**:15, 1973.

Sutton, R. N. P., Marston, S. D., Almond, E. J. P. *et al.*: Asymptomatic infection with EB virus. *J. Clin. Pathol.*, **27**:97, 1974.

Templeton, A. C.: Leukaemia. In: *Tumors in a Tropical Country*, 300 (A. C. Templeton, editor) (Berlin, Heidelberg, New York: Springer-Verlag, 1973).

Tischendorf, P., Shramek, G. J., Balagtas, R. C. *et al.*: Development and persistence of immunity to Epstein–Barr virus in man. *J. Infect. Dis.*, **122**:401, 1970.

Vanier, T. M. and Pike, M. C.: Leukaemia incidence in tropical Africa. *Lancet*, **1**:512, 1967.

Williams, E. H., Day, N. E. and Geser, A. G.: Seasonal variation in onset of Burkitt's lymphoma in the West Nile district of Uganda. *Lancet*, **2**:19, 1974.

Williams, E. H., Spit, P. and Pike, M. C.: Further evidence of space-time clustering of Burkitt's lymphoma in the West Nile district of Uganda. *Brit. J. Cancer*, **23**:235, 1969.

Wright, D. H.: Burkitt's tumor in England. A comparison with childhood lymphosarcoma. *Int. J. Cancer*, **1**:503, 1966.

Zur-Hausen, H.: EBV DNA in biopsies of Burkitt tumors and anaplastic carcinomas of the nasopharynx. *Nature (London)*, **228**:1056, 1970.

Zur-Hausen, H. and Schulte-Holthausen, H.: Presence of EB virus nucleic acid homology in a 'virus free' line of Burkitt tumor cells. *Nature (London)*, **227**:245, 1970.

CHAPTER 4

Other lymphomas

Epidemiologic studies of the non-Hodgkin's lymphomas as one entity, while perhaps a useful first step, have obvious limitations. This is particularly true with regard to attempts to identify aetiologic factors. Clearly there are sufficient differences between reticulum cell sarcoma, lymphosarcoma and Hodgkin's disease to warrant viewing them separately at present. In contrast to Hodgkin's disease, lymphosarcoma and reticulum cell sarcoma are rarely localised (Rosenberg and Kaplar, 1970) have unpredictable patterns of spread and frequently involve tonsillar tissue and extra nodal sites, including the bone marrow and liver (Peters *et al.*, 1968). This latter observation is particularly true of reticulum cell sarcoma. There is a high frequency of gastrointestinal tract involvement in the non-Hodgkin's lymphomas of childhood, and the pattern of spread in Hodgkin's disease seems to be contiguous whereas in these other lymphomas it is non-contiguous. Other important differences relate to complications and response to therapy. Lymphosarcoma is frequently associated with a lymphatic leukaemia stage. This occurs with less frequency with reticulum cell sarcoma and is rare in Hodgkin's disease (Beutler, 1954; Rosenberg *et al.*, 1961). Nitrogen mustard appears to be more effective in Hodgkin's disease than with the other lymphomas, which are in general more resistant to therapy (Livingston and Carter, 1970).

Marked epidemiologic differences between each of the three major lymphomas can also be seen. Although lymphosarcoma and reticulum cell sarcoma are predominantly male disorders, as is Hodgkin's disease, the age specific incidence of these three disorders are different (Mac-Mahon, 1966). Hodgkin's disease has a characteristic bimodal age incidence curve in most countries whereas reticulum cell sarcoma, a lymphomatous process of the elderly, rarely occurs in the young. An observation not fully appreciated at present is that there is evidence to suggest that lymphosarcoma might also be a bimodal disease, with peaks in early childhood (Grundy *et al.*, 1973) and old age.

A subsequent classification of the non-Hodgkin's lymphomas (Table

Table 4.1 Classifications of non-Hodgkin's lymphomas

Previous terminology	Cellular classification	Morphology
Lymphosarcoma ⎱ Giant follicular lymphoma ⎰——>	Lymphocytic (well or poorly differentiated)	diffuse or nodular
Reticulum cell sarcoma ⎱ Giant follicular lymphoma ⎰——>	Histiocytic	diffuse or nodular
Giant follicular lymphoma ⎱——>	Mixed (histiocytic-lympho-cytic)	nodular

4.1) was proposed by Gall and Rappaport (1958) and modified by Berard (1972). A major contribution of this categorisation is that it is based on the major cell type involved in the histologic lesion, be it lymphocytic, histiocytic or undifferentiated. Furthermore, as is true of the Rye classification in Hodgkin's disease, it serves as a fairly accurate prognostic yardstick. A major limitation of this classification is the numerous clinical and histologic variants included under each heading (Table 4.1). As Berard and Dorfman (1974) have pointed out, well-differentiated lymphocytic lymphomas are usually seen in the elderly and frequently represent the tissue manifestation of chronic lymphatic leukaemia. Lesions containing a multiplicity of mature lymphocytes in the young are usually indicative of some reactive process or Hodgkin's disease of the lymphocytic predominant subtype. Marked differences in childhood and adult poorly-differentiated lymphocytic lymphomas have also been observed. Adults frequently present with peripheral lympha-denopathy whereas in children, mediastinal and intra-abdominal sites are common (Rosenberg *et al.*, 1958; Bailey *et al.*, 1961). Histologically, children rarely have a nodular follicular pattern, which is common in adults. Even within the histiocytic lymphomas, we find histiologic vari-ants with divergent characteristics. Leukaemic reticulo-endotheliosis (hairy cell leukaemia) is a chronic slowly progressive disorder charac-terised by hepato-splenomegaly, minimal lymph node involvement, pancytopenia with a relative lymphocytosis, and occasionally neo-plastic cells with cytoplasmic projections in the peripheral blood (Bouroncle *et al.*, 1958). In contrast, histiocytic medullary reticulosis (Scott and Robb-Smith, 1939) is a rapidly fulminant disorder with hepato-splenomegaly and progressive pancytopenia.

As our knowledge of various aspects of the malignant lymphomas increases, histological classifications must accordingly be modified or changed. In recent years, there have been rapid advances in the field of immunology, particularly with respect to the primary lymphoreticular disorders. Stated simply, we now realise that all lymphocytes are not the same, that thymic (T) and bursal (B) cells each undergo several stages of development, and that the number and type of lymphocytes may vary with age and sex. These observations are bound to have a profound effect on our future understanding of lymphoreticular malignancies and it seems quite possible, considering the heterogeneity of the lymphocyte population in both type and developmental stage, that there may be many more variations in the lymphomas than has been appreciated. This poses a great challenge to both the pathologist and immunologist for what is required is a classification which merges histology (general morphology and descriptive cell type) with current immunologic theory. T-cell disorders are thought to involve primarily interfollicular zones and include Hodgkin's disease (Gergley *et al.*, 1973; Grifoni *et al.*, 1972), certain acute lymphatic leukaemias (Chin *et al.*, 1973) including Sternberg sarcoma (Smith *et. al.*, 1973) mycoses fungoides, Sezary's syndrome and possibly a minority of cases of chronic lymphatic leukaemia (Seligmann *et al.*, 1973). B-cell disorders, which are thought to effect mainly follicular centres, include most chronic lymphatic leukaemia cases, lymphoblastic lymphomas, Burkitt's lymphoma and reticulum cell or histiocytic sarcomas (Frøland *et al.*, 1972; Aisenberg and Bloch, 1972, Seligmann *et al.*, 1973). While this immunologic categorisation is preliminary, and it may well be that the T and B systems are interrelated in a highly integrated fashion (e.g. a B-cell disorder might be due to a defect in the T system or both), it does represent an additional dimension in our understanding of the lymphoreticular disorders. Using these immunologic concepts, we can also attempt to understand possible interrelationships between certain diseases. Is mycosis fungoides the adult counterpart of childhood lymphatic leukaemia with a mediastinal mass? Patients with Sezary's syndrome may develop malignant lymphomas with both cutaneous and visceral involvement. Is this disorder a variant of mycosis fungoides? It has long been appreciated that lymphosarcoma and chronic lymphatic leukaemia can co-exist (Rappaport, 1964) and that the postmortem appearance of these two diseases can be quite similar. If both are disorders of the same immune pathway and perhaps related, there must be some explanation for the relatively high incidence of lymphosarcoma in far eastern countries when compared with chronic lymphatic leukaemia rates (Anderson *et al.*, 1970).

AETIOLOGIC CLUES

The immunologic surveillance theory of Burnet (1967) postulates that during the life of an organism, transformed cells are continually appearing, but these cells can not proliferate because of an immune mechanism which recognises them as foreign. According to this theory then the development of a tumour would be indicative of some failure in the cellular immune mechanism responsible for rejection. It has also been proposed that immunostimulation might result in neoplastic transformation (Fialkow, 1967; Prehn and Lappe, 1971), a concept that is supported by the observation that an immune response can be associated with more efficient tumour growth than would occur in the absence of such a reaction (Prehn, 1972). Thus, a weak but persistent antigenic stimulus might enhance tumour growth, whereas a strong one might inhibit this transformation. These theories suggest that some aberration in the host immune system might be essential for the development of certain lymphomas and it seems possible that both a persistent antigenic stimulation and an immune suppressed host might be required. Antigenic stimulation can result from a variety of factors especially infections due to slow viruses, immunosuppression by radio or chemotherapy, immune deficiency states, inherited or acquired and chronic infection (Bellanti, 1972). In Burkitt's lymphoma (Chapter 3), the Epstein–Barr virus and chronic malaria have been thought to be important antigenic and/or immunosuppressive agents. Primary intestinal lymphoma with malabsorption is another example of a lymphoreticular malignancy in which some form of chronic antigenic stimulation is thought to be required. This syndrome is common in Israel and Arab countries (Ramot and Many, 1972), but rare in Western countries (Edelman *et al.*, 1966). In Israel it is relatively prevalent in Arabs and first and second generation Jewish immigrants from mideastern and North African countries, but extremely rare among Jews of European ancestry. In children, a solitary lymphoma of the ileum is usually found whereas in adults, involvement of the small intestine is usually diffuse. Histologically this lymphoma is usually histiocytic in type. Another syndrome characterised by malabsorption, lymphocytic infiltration of the intestine and a fragment of IgA heavy chain in the serum has also been described (Seligmann *et al.*, 1968) and this may be a variant of the histiocytic lymphoma syndrome. In the United States, where intestinal lymphomas are quite rare, there is evidence to suggest an association with prior coeliac sprue (Harris *et al.*, 1967). This does not appear to be true in Israel or Arabian countries where it has been suggested that intestinal parasitism in under privileged populations might serve as an antigenic stimulus. Long-term epidemiologic studies of patients with malabsorption and heavy chain IgA are needed to further evaluate their possible association with primary intestinal lymphomas. In addition to the examples mentioned, there is evidence, both epidemiologic and experimental, to suggest the potentially important role of immunosuppression in the development of malignant lymphomas. Several reports have documented an increased frequency of malignancies, particularly reticulum cell sarcoma, in organ homograft recipients (Doll and Kinlen, 1970; Hoover and Fraumeni, 1973) receiving immunosuppresive therapy (azathioprine or antilymphocyte serum). Recent evidence further suggests that this lymphoma arises from host, not donor cells (Brown *et al.*, 1974). These observations are of great importance for they provided the basis for several important questions. Why should there be a 350-fold increased risk of reticulum cell sarcoma? In contrast to other post-transplant cancers (e.g. brain, liver and skin cancer) where the risk apparently increases with time, the excess lymphoma risk appears within a year of transplantation and apparently remains at the same high level thereafter. Is this due to a defect in suppressor T-cell function resulting in incomplete regulation of lymphocyte proliferation or does immunosuppression set the stage for a subsequent or latent viral induced lymphoreticular malignancy? Available experimental evidence would appear to support the second hypothesis, for in certain animals an increased incidence of viral induced tumours, especially leukaemias and lymphomas, occur after thymectomy or the administration of prednisone or antilymphocyte serum (Doell *et al.*, 1967; Casey, 1968; Starzel *et al.*, 1971). Furthermore, Hirsh *et al.* (1972) have demonstrated that lymphoid cells participating in a graft vs. host reaction allow activation and release of latent viruses oncogenic for lymphoid tissue. A great deal of information might be obtained by conducting controlled retrospective epidemiologic and prospective sero-epidemiologic studies on organ transplant candidates. In addition to the above considerations, another intriguing observation is the rarity of Hodgkin's disease in the immunosuppressed transplant patient. This suggests that although cellular anergy can occur in advanced stages of this disorder, prior immunosuppression, as determined by available immunologic tests, may not be an essential factor. While the studies of Young *et al.*, (1972) are consistent with this suggestion, the matter is far from settled. A recent study of cellular immunity in Hodgkin's disease (Winkelstein *et al.*, 1974) suggests that neither skin test reactivity nor the response to phytohaemagglutinin fully assess the status of cell-mediated immunity in patients with Hodgkin's disease. New probes might be required to detect important alterations in immunologic responses to this disorder.

There is still further evidence which supports the concept that some alteration in host immunity might be a prerequisite for the development of certain lymphomas. Inherited immune deficiency conditions, such as the Chediak–Higashi, Wiskot–Aldrich, and ataxia-telangiectasia syndromes (Chapter 7) are associated with an increased incidence of lymphomas. Furthermore, there may be an association between lympho-reticular malignancy and certain auto-immune disorders. The strongest relationship appears to be between Sjögren's syndrome (Mikulicz disease) and the development of lymphomas. It is also interesting to note that there appears to be an increased frequency of auto-antibodies, especially of the smooth muscle type of cancer patients (Farrow *et al.*, 1970). Talal and his colleagues (1964, 1967, 1970) have described several instances of reticulum cell sarcoma developing in patients with Sjögren's syndrome. Azzopardi and Evans (1971) reported five additional instances of lymphoma complicating Mikulicz disease (without rheumatoid arthritis). The most intriguing features of these five cases were: they all had histologic evidence of benign lympho-epithelial lesions in their salivary glands and either simultaneously or at a later date of a malignant lymphoma; three patients developed Hodgkin's disease and the others, recticulum cell sarcoma; and in all instances these lymphomas developed in the same anatomic site where Mikulicz disease was present. As these authors point out, however, the precise relationship of the two processes is uncertain; the possibilities that must be considered are: that the lymphoma might have led to the development of the lympho–epithelial lesions observed, that these lesions may in fact progress to a malignant lymphoma or that both diseases may be expressions of the same underlying defect. An interesting feature of Sjögren's syndrome is that impaired cellular immunity is frequently present in patients with this disorder (Whaley *et al.*, 1970). Other reports have suggested that an association may exist between malignant lymphomas and prior rheumatic disease, Hashimoto's thyroiditis, lupus erythematosis, adult dermatomyositis, idiopathic steatorrhea (Azzopardi and Evans, 1971; Cox, 1964; Williams, 1959; Hargraves, 1962; Cammarata *et al.*, 1963) and it has been shown that in mice auto-immune haemolytic anaemia frequently precedes the development of certain malignant lymphomas (Mellors, 1966). However, detailed epidemiologic studies, employing objective diagnostic criteria, will be required to properly evaluate the possibility that some relationship exists between these disorders and the subsequent development of certain lymphomas. In designing such studies, attention should also be given to other possible auto-immune diseases. These include pernicious anaemia, Addison's disease, lupoid hepatitis, idiopathic thrombocytopenic purpura, regional enteritis, ulcerative colitis, coeliac syndrome, sprue and eczema. Furthermore, special consideration should be given to the possibility that an auto-immune syndrome may represent a complication of an underlying lymphoreticular disorder, especially lymphosarcoma and chronic lymphatic leukaemia. It is also important to realise that a homogenous monoclonal immunoglobulin elevation, while present in patients with multiple myeloma, macroglobulinaemia and some cases of chronic lymphatic leukaemia, may also occur in patients with no evidence of these disorders or with some chronic infection (Morgenfeld, 1974). This example is provided to emphasise the caution required in interpreting laboratory studies, and the need for histologic confirmation of all diagnosis. Despite the confusion surrounding the relationship between malignant lymphomas and prior auto-immune disorders, it is important that future studies be conducted in this area. In addition to the clinical evidence suggesting an association, Schwartz and Beldotti (1965) reported the induction of lymphomas in animals by graft–host reactions.

Some mention has already been made about the pharmacological agents capable of suppressing host immunity. There is additional indirect evidence suggesting a possible association between chemical exposure and the subsequent development of lymphoreticular malignancies. A higher than expected frequency of lymphomas has been reported among chemists (Li *et al.*, 1969), anaesthesiologists (Bruce *et al.*, 1968) and patients receiving certain anticonvulsant drugs (Saltzstein and Ackerman, 1959). It is also known that chemicals, such as certain polycyclic hydrocarbons can induce lymphomas in mice (Pietra *et al.*, 1959). A recent case–control study has suggested that the prior use of amphetamines might predispose to Hodgkin's disease (Newall *et al.*, 1973). All of these considerations merit further evaluation. This is particularly true of the possible aetiologic role of the hydantoin drugs in Hodgkin's disease and other malignant lymphomas (Saltzstein *et al.*, 1958; 1959; Saltzstein, 1962). Since Saltzstein *et al.* (1958) reported a case of a Hodgkin's like disease in an epileptic patient receiving a hydantoin derivative, several additional cases have been reported (Gams *et al.*, 1968; Hyman and Sommers, 1966). Although in most instances the signs of lymphoma disappeared after therapy with this agent was discontinued, in some regression did not occur. Despite the fact that a causal association with certain lymphomas is not established at present, it seems clear that hydantoin derivatives can induce certain lympho-proliferative reactions. These include reticulum cell hyperplasia, eosinophilia, lymphatic hyperplasia, an increase in plasma cells and occasionally Reed–Sternberg-like cells. Furthermore, there have been reports of true lymphomas occurring in epileptic patients who received hydantoin drugs. Hyman and Sommers (1966) reported seven cases, four with Hodgkin's disease and three with lymphosarcoma. Most of the patients had been treated with hydantoin drugs for long periods, as much as fifteen years, before they presented with malignant lymphomas and the discontinuation of anticonvulsant therapy had no apparent effect on the progress of the lymphoma. Other studies suggesting an association between hydantoin therapy and various lymphoreticular malignancies have been reviewed in a *Lancet* editorial (1971). If these observations are indicative of a real association, what might be the nature of this relationship? It seems possible that certain hydantoin drugs might be able to induce a malignant state either directly or indirectly through some influence on the immune system. In favour of this latter hypothesis is the fact that hypo- and hyper-gammaglobu-linaemia plasma cell dyscrasias and red blood cell aplasia (Jeong *et al.*, 1974) have been associated with these drugs.

Radiation represents yet another well-established cause of immuno-suppression, and there is some evidence suggesting an association between prior exposure and the development of certain lymphoreticular disorders. An increased frequency of malignant lymphomas and multiple myeloma (Nishiyama *et al.*, 1973) has been reported among survivors of the atomic bomb in Hiroshima exposed to 100 rad or more, especially if they were exposed when less than twenty-five years of age. Although a similar association was not found in Nagasaki, the possibility has been raised that this may have been due to a different radiation spectrum emitted by the two bombs or biological differences between the inhabi-tants of the two areas. Although not established, if such a relationship were confirmed it would not be surprising for both T- and B-lympho-cytes are radiosensitive (Wood *et al.*, 1974). Considering the possibility that T-lymphocytes in the irradiated patient might remain suppressed for longer periods than B-lymphocytes (Wood *et al.*, 1974), it would be interesting to know what specific types of malignant lymphomas were most prevalent in Hiroshima.

Up to this point, the major emphasis has been placed on those factors which can alter host immunity and possibly enhance the development of lymphoreticular malignancies. This must be considered a central theme with respect to certain lymphomas, since all available evidence suggests that the major immunologic defence against these disorders appears to be cell-mediated. The possible importance of humoural factors must be explored in further detail. Table 4.2 summarises some of the immunologic responses found in certain neoplastic disorders of the reticulo-endothelial system. The challenge that these observations define can be stated briefly: what factors, in addition to those described, are capable of diminishing the ability of the host's immune system to ward off neoplastic growth. They may vary both in type and relative importance in different regions of the world. Particular attention should be given to pharmacologic agents in developed countries for it has become increasingly apparent that no drug is without its side effects. Even the ingestion of aspirin, one of the most benign drugs, might be associated with suppressed lymphocyte transformation (Chimel, 1973).

VIRUSES AND LYMPHORETICULAR MALIGNANCIES

The possible role of viruses as co-factors (e.g. Burkitt's lymphoma) or in the production of auto-immunity has already been mentioned. Viruses with a cell-transforming capacity might also play a role in the induction of certain lymphomas because of their immunosuppressive capacities (Ceglowski and Friedman, 1968; Wedderburn and Salanar, 1968). Thus, even if there is a real causal association between infection and lymphoma development, it may be sufficient but not essential in nature. However, there is experimental evidence that certain DNA and RNA viruses alone are capable of inducing lymphoreticular malignancy (Table 4.3). In animal tumours caused by RNA viruses, reproduction and release of new viruses may not be associated with damage to host cells whereas the DNA oncogenic viruses are lytic. Infection with the RNA oncornaviruses is thought therefore to result in a steady state with essentially transformed host cells (Allen and Cole, 1972; Pasqualini and Caparo, 1974). This group of viruses has several additional important characteristics; they are fairly widespread in animal populations, and are known causes of tumours in vertebrates and may produce disease

Table 4.2   Immunologic responses in reticulo-endothelial neoplasia

Immunologic reaction	Type of neoplasia				
	Hodgkin's	Acute leukaemia	Chronic lymphocytic leukaemia	Multiple myeloma	Lymphosarcoma and reticulum cell sarcoma
Skin-delayed hypersensitivity	Impaired to absent; no relationship with progression or duration but restored in remission	Intact except in lymphocytopenia	Established: intact New: impaired to absent	Established: intact New: impaired	Impaired
Skin allograft	Prolonged rejection		Normal or prolonged	Prolonged rejection	Prolonged rejection Impaired
Lymphocyte transformation	Impaired to absent Restored in remission Serum factor impairs normal cell blastogenesis Restored with normal RNA Antilymphocyte absent		Impaired or delayed	Normal PHA(?), impaired to absent to Ag	
Passive transfer of delayed hypersensitivity by cells	Unsuccessful 0/9 1/22		Successful		
Ab formation (primary)	Variable, little clinical data Mumps CF normal Typhoid aggl. normal Tularaemia impaired to absent Pneum. polysaccharide impaired to absent Normal	Intact	Primary impaired	Primary impaired Secondary low	Primary impaired Secondary impaired
Complement	Restored in remission; impaired to absent				
Phagocytosis periph		Inconclusive but probably impaired	Impaired (?) restored by normal serum		
R-E fixed I clearance	Increased	Abnormal		Variable	Normal

Table 4.3   DNA and RNA viruses that are oncogenic for certain experimental animals

Type of virus RNA Oncornaviruses (leukoviruses)	
Type C	leukaemia (avian, feline, murine, hamster)
	sarcoma (avian, feline, murine)
Type B	murine mammary tumour
DNA	
Herpes	Marek's disease
	Lucké renal-carcinoma
	Herpes sylvilagus
	Herpes saimiri
	Herpes ateles
	Epstein–Barr virus
	Herpes hominis (simplex) types 1 and 2
Adenovirus	Types 3, 7, 12, 14, 16, 18, 21, 31
Papova	Polyoma
	Papilloma
	Vacuolating

only after long latent periods. Of great importance is the observation that infection usually occurs during the fetal period. In cats, however, who have the highest incidence of lymphomas among mammals (Dorn *et al.*, 1967) there is good evidence that horizontal transmission of feline leukaemia virus occurs (Jarrett *et al.*, 1973). Interestingly, although the alimentary form is the most common type of feline lymphoma, in young cats the anterior mediastinal location is most frequent.

Of the various oncogenic DNA viruses, herpes viruses have been the most associated with lymphoreticular malignancies (Allen and Cole, 1972; Pasqualini and Caparo, 1974). Marek's disease, a lymphoma of chickens is caused by a herpes virus. In contrast to lymphoid leukosis, a closely related disorder which occurs at an older age and produces intrafollicular lesions, Marek's disease occurs in younger chickens and is interfollicular (Churchill, 1968). Herpes saimiri and ateles can produce lymphatic leukaemia and lymphoma in owl monkeys and marmosets (Melendez *et al.*, 1971; 1972). It is interesting that the incubation period can vary from as little as three days to more than 200 days with these agents. The evidence associating the Epstein–Barr virus with Burkitt's lymphoma has already been presented. Characteristic features that most of the herpes viruses seem to have in common are ubiquity, latency and a low degree of virulence. With the possible exception of Burkitt's lymphoma, there is no evidence implicating a specific viral agent in the aetiology of any human lymphoma. C-type particles have been observed in certain human lymphomas (Dmochowski, 1970) and virus-like agents have been reported in cultures prepared from Hodgkin's tissue (Eisinger *et al.*, 1971), but as yet no causative association has been established.

How should these observations be viewed? Admittedly they do not provide any clear-cut evidence as to the aetiology of the various lympho-proliferative malignancies in man, but it must be realised that they represent a great potential source for hypotheses which might prove to be highly relevant to the situation in humans. In addition there are certain general features of certain animal models which might be applicable to these disorders in man. A characteristic feature of many of the oncogenic animal viruses is latency; in man this might be reflected by a long incubation period. This possibility and the evidence suggesting that some prior aberration in the host's immune system might be required for certain lymphomas to occur, suggests that if any of these disorders can be caused by viruses, they are not contagious in the manner influenza is. Even in certain viral induced neoplasia in lower animals, a certain underlying susceptibility must be present. This may be genetic (McDevitt, 1971), immunologic (Hays, 1972) or both. Animal studies also indicate that age and time of exposure may be important factors. The epidemiologist who employs a time–space cluster analysis to evaluate the possibility that person-to-person transmission or some common exposure occurs in a disease, must therefore look for the most likely co-ordinates. He must also realise that negative results might be indicative only of the fact that the wrong ones were selected. Another important consideration relates to the mode of transmission. Cat leukaemia can be transmitted to other cats vertically and horizontally. Horizontal transmission occurs among chickens with Marek's disease. There is no evidence to suggest that avian leukoses viruses infect mammals but the cat sarcoma virus is transmissible to primates. Two basic questions emerge from these observations. If certain oncogenic viruses are capable of crossing the species barrier, to what extent might they affect man? Secondly, it seems possible that both vertical and horizontal transmission might occur in certain lymphoproliferative malignancies, especially those characterised by childhood and adult age incidence peaks; thus in the young it might be chiefly vertical whereas in the elderly, horizontal transmission might predominate. In certain childhood lymphomas, the demonstration of seasonality by birth month might provide important results, especially if it were shown to vary concomitantly with the activity of a specific viral disease. Case-control studies of antecedent exposure are applicable to both childhood and adult lymphoid disorders. In this type of study, however, great care must be employed in selecting the proper controls and probably several different ones should be used. Another method of evaluating common exposure or person–to–person transmission in young adults and older cases is the index-secondary case approach. This design is particularly useful in institutions, such as schools, where the population at risk is well-defined.

Familial studies are also of some value, especially if factors such as the time and age intervals between diagnosis and the proximity of related cases are all considered. While this approach has certain limitations, it is also useful in determining whether relatives of cases with lymphoreticular disorders have an increased risk of developing these disorders and if so, the specific types. A study of this type was conducted by Rosenlot *et al.*, (1971) (Table 4.4), but further investigation along these lines is required.

Table 4.4 **Disease interrelationships noted in Central Nebraska multiple-case family study (February 1970; 55 families).** (From: Rosenlof, R. C.; Lemon, H. M. and Rigby, P. G. (1971), by courtesy of *National Cancer Institute Monograph.*)

Diagnosis of proband	Number of probands	Diagnosis most frequent in relatives	Total relatives with disease diagnosis
(a) Lymphosarcoma or lymphoma, unspecified	10	Acute lymphatic leukaemia	5
(b) Hodgkin's disease, giant follicular lymphoma	10	Hodgkin's disease	12
(c) Chronic lymphocytic leukaemia	9	Acute lymphatic leukaemia Chronic lymphocytic leukaemia	6
(d) Acute lymphatic leukaemia	8	Acute lymphatic leukaemia	21
(e) Acute myelogenous leukaemia	4	Acute lymphatic leukaemia	2
(f) Chronic myelogenous leukaemia	4	—	1
(g) Multiple myeloma	4	—	2
(h) Reticulum cell sarcoma	3	—	0

References

Aisenberg, A. C. and Bloch, K.: Immunoglobulins on the surface of neoplastic lymphocytes. *New Eng. J. Med.*, **287**:272, 1972.

Allen, D. W. and Cole, P.: Viruses and human cancer. *New Eng. J. Med.*, **286**:70, 1972.

Anderson, R. E., Ishida, K., Li, Y. *et al.*: Geographic aspects of malignant lymphoma and multiple myeloma. *Amer. J. Pathol.*, **61**:85, 1970.

Azzopardi, J. G. and Evans, D. J.: Malignant lymphoma of parotid associated with Mikulicz disease (benign lymphoepithelial lesion). *J. Clin. Pathol.*, **24**:744, 1971.

Bailey, R. J., Burgert, E. D. and Dahlin, D. C.: Malignant lymphoma in children. *Pediat.*, **28**;985, 1961.

Bellanti, J. A.: Suppression of the immune response. In: *Immunology* 160 (Philadelphia, London, Toronto: W. B. Saunders Co., 1972).

Berard, C. W.: Histopathology of lymphoreticular disorders. In: *Hematology*, 901 (W. J. Williams, editor), (New York: McGraw-Hill, 1972).

Berard, C. W. and Dorfman, R. F.: Histopathology of malignant lymphomas. In: *Clinics in Hematology*, 3 (S. A., Rosenberg, editor), (London, Philadelphia, Toronto: W. B. Saunders Co, 1974, 39).

Beutler, E.: The development of acute myelogenous leukemia in a patient with reticulum cell lymphoma. *Ann. Int. Med.*, **40**:1217, 1954.

Bouroncle, B. A. Wiseman, B. K. and Doan, C. A.: Leukemic reticuloendotheliosis. *Blood*, **13**:609, 1958.

Brown, R. C., Schiff, M. and Mitchell, M. S.: Reticulum cell sarcoma of host origin arising in a transplanted kidney. *Ann. Int. Med.*, **80**:459, 1974.

Bruce, D. L., Eide, K. A., Linde, H. W. *et al.*: Causes of death among anesthesiologists: a 20 year survey. *Anesthesiology*, **29**:565, 1968.

Burnet, F. M.: Immunologic aspects of malignant disease. *Lancet*, **1**:1171, 1967.

Cammarata, R. J., Rodman, G. P. and Jensen, W. N.: Systemic rheumatic disease and malignant lymphoma. *Arch. Int. Med.*, **111**:330, 1963.

Casey, T. P.: The development of lymphomas in mice with autoimmune disorders treated with azathioprine. *Blood*, **31**:396, 1968.

Ceglowski, W. S. and Friedman, H.: Immunosuppressive effects of Friend and Rauscher leukemia disease viruses on cellular and humoral antibody formation. *J. Nat. Cancer Inst.*, **40**:983, 1968.

Chimel, H.: Suppression of lymphocyte transformation by aspirin. *Lancet*, **2**:861, 1973.

Chin, A. H., Saiki, J. H., Trujillo, J. M. *et al.*: Periferal blood T and B lymphocytes in patients with lymphoma and acute leukemia. *Clin. Immunol. Immunopathol.*, **1**:499, 1973.

Churchill, A. E.: Herpes-type virus isoloated in cell culture from tumors of chickens with Marek's disease: I. studies in cell culture, *J. Nat. Cancer Inst.*, **41**:939, 1968.

Cox, M. T.: Malignant lymphoma of thyroid. *J. Clin. Pathol.*, **17**:591, 1964.

Dmochowski, L.: Current status of the relationship of viruses to leukemia, lymphoma, and solid tumors, in Leukemia-Lymphoma. A collection of papers presented at the 14th. *Annual Clinical Conference on Cancer, 1969, at the University of Texas*, 37 (Chicago: Year Book Med. Pub., 1970).

Doell, R. G., DeVaux St. Cyr., C. and Graber, P.: Immune reactivity prior to development of thymic lymphoma in C57BL mice. *Int. J. Cancer*, **2**:103, 1967.

Doll, R. and Kinlen, L.: Immunosurveillance and cancer: epidemiological evidence. *Brit. Med. J.*, 4:420, 1970.

Dorn, C. R., Taylor, D. O. N. and Gibbard, H. H.: Epizoetiologic characteristics of canine and feline leukemia and lymphoma. *Amer. J. Vet. Res.*, 28:993, 1967.

Edelman, S., Parkins, R. A. and Rubin, C. E.: Abdominal lymphoma presenting as malabsorption. *Medicine*, 45:111, 1966.

Eisinger, M., Fox, S. M., DeHarven, E. *et al.*: Virus-like agent from patients with Hodgkin's disease. *Nature (London)*, 233:104, 1971.

Farrow, L. J., Holborow, E. J., Johnson, G. D. *et al.*: Autoantibodies and hepatitis associated antigen in acute infective hepatitis. *Brit. Med. J.*, 2:693, 1970.

Fialkow, P. J.: Hypothesis: 'Immunologic oncogenesis'. *Blood*, 30:388, 1967.

Froland, S. S., Natvig, J. B. and Stavem, P.: Immunologic characterization of lymphocytes in lymphoproliferative disorders. Restriction of classes, subclasses and allotypes of membrane-bound Ig. *Scand. J. Immunol.*, 1:351, 1972.

Gall, E. A. and Rappaport, H.: Seminar on diseases of lymph nodes and spleen. In: *Proceedings of the 23rd Seminar of the American Society of Clinical Pathology*, 1 (J. R., MacDonald, editor) (Amer. Soc. Clin. Pathol., 1951).

Gams, R. A., Neal, J. A. and Conrad, F. G.: Hydantoin induced pseudolymphoma. *Ann. Int. Med.*, 69:557, 1968.

Gergely, P., Szegedi, G., Berenyl, E. *et al.*: Lymphocyte surface immunoglobulins in Hodgkin's disease. *New Eng. J. Med.*, 289:220, 1973.

Grifoni, V., DelGiaco, G. S., Manconi, P.E. *et al.*: Surface immunoglobulins in lymphocytes in Hodgkin's disease. *Lancet*, 1:848, 1972.

Grundy, G. W., Creagen, E. T. and Fraumeni, J. F.: Non-Hodgkin's lymphoma in childhood: epidemiologic features. *J. Nat. Cancer Inst.*, 51: 767, 1973.

Hargraves, M. M.; Leukemia and the G.P. *J. Arkansas Med. Soc.*, 58:522, 1962.

Harris, O. D., Cooke, W. T., Thompson, H. *et al.*: Malignancy in adult coeliac disease and idiopathic steatorrhoea. *Amer. J. Med.*, 42:899, 1967.

Hays, E. F.: Graft-versus-host reactions and the viral induction of mouse lymphoma. *Cancer Res.*, 32:270, 1972.

Hirsch, M. S., Phillips, S. M., Solnick, C. *et al.*: Activation of leukemia virus by graft-versus-host and mixed lymphocyte reactions *in vitro. Proceedings of the National Acad. of Sci. of the USA*, 69:1069, 1972.

Hoover, R. and Fraumeni, J. F.: Risk of cancer in renal transplant recipients. *Lancet*, 2:55, 1973.

Hyman, G. and Sommers, S.: The development of Hodgkin's disease and other lymphomas during anticonvulsant therapy. *Blood*, 28:416, 1966.

Jarrett, W., Jarrett, O., Lindsay, M. *et al.*,: Horizontal transmission of leukemia virus and leukemia in the cat. *J. Nat. Cancer Inst.*, 51:833, 1973.

Jeong, Y. G., Jung, Y. and River, G. L.: Pure RBC aplasia and diphenylhydantoin. *J.A.M.A.*, 229:314, 1974.

Lancet, editorial: Is phenytoin carcinogenic? 2:1071, 1971.

Li, F. Fraumeni, J. F., Mantel, N. *et al.*: Cancer mortality among chemists. *J. Nat. Cancer Inst.*, 43:1159, 1969.

Livingstone, R. B. and Carter, S. K.: Single Agents in Cancer Chemotherapy, I (New York: Plenum Publishing Corp, 1970).

MacMahon, B.: Epidemiology of Hodgkin's disease. *Cancer Res.*, 26:1189, 1966.

McDevitt, H. O.: Relationship between histocompatibility antigens and immune response. *Transplant Proc.*, 3:1321, 1971.

Melendez, L. V., Hunt, R. D., Daniel, M. D. *et al.*: Acute lymphocytic leukemia in owl monkeys inoculated with Herpes virus saimiri. *Science*, **171**:1161, 1971.

Melendez, L. V., Hunt, R. D., Daniel, M. D., *et al.*: Herpes viruses saimiri and ateles their role in malignant lymphomas of monkeys. *Fed. Proc.*, **31**:1643, 1972.

Mellors, R. C.: Autoimmune disease in NZB/BL mice II. Autoimmunity and malignant lymphoma. *Blood*, **27**:435, 1966.

Morgenfeld, M. C.: Toxoplasmosis. *Medicina*, **34**:48, 1974.

Newall, G. R., Rawlings, W., Kinnear, B. K. *et al.*: Case-control study of Hodgkin's disease I. Results of the interview questionnaire. *J. Nat. Cancer Inst.*, **51**:1437, 1973.

Nishiyama, H., Anderson, R. E., Ishimaru, T. *et al.*: The incidence of malignant lymphoma and multiple myeloma in Hiroshima and Nagasaki atomic bomb survivors. *Cancer*, **32**:1301, 1973.

Pasqualini, C. D. and Caparo, A. C.: Zoonosis and its possible relation with lymphoma and leukemia in man. *Medicina*, **34**:1, 1974.

Peters, M. V., Hasselback, R. and Brown, T. C.: The natural history of the lymphomas related to clinical classification. In: *Proceedings of the International Conference on Leukemia-Lymphoma*, 357 (C. J. D. Zarafonetis, editor) (Philadelphia: Lea and Febiger, 1968).

Pietra, G., Spencer, K. and Shubik, P.: Response of newly born mice to a chemical carcinogen. *Nature*, *(London)*, **183**:1689, 1959.

Prehn, R. T.: The immune reaction as a stimulator of tumor growth. *Science*, **176**:170, 1972.

Prehn, R. and Lappe, M. A.: An immunostimulation theory of tumor develoment. *Transplant Rev.*, **7**:26, 1971.

Ramot, B. and Many, A.: Primary intestinal lymphoma: clinical manifestations and possible effect of environmental factors. In: *Current Problems in the Epidemiology of Cancer and Lymphomas*, 193 (E. Grundmann and H. Tullinius, editors) (Berlin, Heidelberg, New York: Springer-Verlag, 1972).

Rappaport, H.: The histologic aspects of lymphoreticular neoplasms. In: *Symposium on Lymphoreticular Tumors in Africa*, 174 (F. C. Roulet, editor) (Basel, New York: S. Karger, 1964).

Rosenberg, S. A., Diamond, H. D. and Craver, L. F.: Lymphosarcoma: the effect of therapy and survival in 1,269 patients in a review of 30 years experience. *Medicine*, **40**:31, 1961.

Rosenberg, S. A., Diamond, H. D. and Dargeon, H. W.: Lymphosarcoma in childhood. *New Eng. J. Med.*, **259**:505, 1958.

Rosenberg, S. A. and Kaplan, H. S.: Hodgkin's disease and other malignant lymphomas. *Calif. Med.*, **113**:1970.

Rosenlof, R. C., Lemon, H. M. and Rigby, P. G.: Familial factors relating to prognosis of leukemia and lymphoma. *National Cancer Institute Monograph*, **34**:283, 1971.

Saltzstein, S. L.: Lymphoma or drug reaction occurring during hydantoin therapy for epilepsy. *Amer. J. Med.*, **32**:286, 1962.

Saltzstein, S. L. and Ackerman, L. V.: Lymphadenopathy induced by anticonvulsant drugs and mimicking clinically and pathologically malignant lymphomas. *Cancer*, **12**:164, 1959.

Saltzstein, S. L., Jaudon, J. C., Luse, S. A. *et al.*: Lymphadenopathy induced by ethotoin. Clinical and pathological mimicking of malignant lymphoma. *J.A.M.A.*, **167**:1618, 1958.

Schwartz, R. S. and Beldotti, L:. Malignant lymphomas following allogenic disease: Transition from an immunologic to a neoplastic disorder. *Science*, **149**:1511, 1965.

Scott, R. B. and Robb-Smith, A. H. T.: Histiocytic medullary reticulosis. *Lancet*, **2**:194, 1939.

Seligmann, M., Danon, F. and Hurez, D.: Alpha chain disease: a new immunoglobin abnormality. *Science*, **162**:1396, 1968.

Seligmann, M., Preud Homme, J. L. and Broulet, J. C.: B and T cell markers in human proliferative blood diseases and primary immunodeficiencies with special reference to membrane bound immunoglobulins. *Transpl. Rev* **16**:85, 1973.

Smith, J. L.: Characterization of malignant mediastinal lymphoid neoplasm (Sternberg sarcoma) as thymic in origin. *Lancet*, **1**:74, 1973.

Starzel, T. E., Penn, I., Putnam, C. *et al.*: Iatrogenic allergy of immunologic surveillance in man and their influence on malignancies. *Transpl. Rev.*, **7**:112, 1971.

Talal, N., Asofsky and Lightbudy, P.: Immunoglobulin synthesis by salivary gland lymphoid cells in Sjögren's syndrome. *J. Clin. Invest.*, **49**:49, 1970.

Talal, N. and Bunin, J. J.: The development of malignant lymphoma in the course of Sjögren's syndrome. *Amer. J. Med.*, **36**:529, 1964.

Talal, N., Sokolov, L. and Bath, W. F.: Extra salivary lymphoid abnormalities in Sjögren's syndrome. *Amer. J. Med.*, **43**:50, 1967.

Wedderburn, N. and Salaman, M. H.: The immunodepressive effect of Friend virus. II. Reduction of splenic hemolysin-producing cells in primary and secondary responses. *Immunology*, **15**:439, 1968.

Whaley, K., Glenn, A. C. A., Dick, W. C. *et al.*: Delayed hypersensitivity in Sjögrens syndrome and rheumatoid arthritis in impaired cell mediated hypersensitivity in man. *Third Symposium of the Charles Salt Research Center*, 25 (J. F. Jennings and D. J. Ward (editors), 1970).

Williams, R. C.: Dermato-myositis and malignancy: a review of the literature. *Ann. Int. Med.*, **50**:1174, 1959.

Winkelstein, A., Mikulla, J. M., Sartiano *et al.*: Cellular immunity in Hodgkin's disease: comparison of cutaneous reactivity and lymphoproliferative response to phytohemagglutinin. *Cancer*, **34**:549 1974.

Wood, S. E., Campbell, J. B., Anderson, J. M. *et al.*: Lymphocyte response after radiotherapy. *Lancet*, **1**:863, 1974.

Young, R. C., Corder, M. P., Haynes, H. A. *et al.*: Delayed hypersensitivity in Hodgkin's disease. *Amer. J. Med.*, **52**:63, 1972.

CHAPTER 5

Acute lymphatic leukaemia in childhood

It has long been appreciated that certain types of acute leukaemia in man might have a viral aetiology, a possibility that is enhanced by various experimental observations in lower animals (Gross, 1961, Epstein 1971). For the most part epidemiologic investigations of human leukaemia have been of two types: descriptive studies and time–space cluster analyses. It is unfortunate, however, that few cluster studies have considered possible differences in histologic subtype, age, seasonality and urban–rural factors. The potential importance of these factors in acute lymphatic leukaemia of childhood is discussed in this chapter and a hypothesis concerning the possible aetiology of this disorder is suggested.

ACUTE LYMPHATIC LEUKAEMIA IN CHILDHOOD—A DISTINCT ENTITY

The fact that each pathologic variety of leukaemia has its own distinct age–specific incidence curve suggests that each subtype might differ aetiologically. Both the lymphatic and myeloid types of chronic leukaemia are rare in childhood (Court Brown et al., 1964) and become progressively more common up to the age of 80 years. In contrast the acute leukaemias are relatively common in childhood (Figure 5.1), but a peak in the 0–4-year age group is limited to the lymphatic type (Court Brown et al., 1964; MacMahon and Clark, 1956). Another difference is that the decrease in incidence after 9 years of age is sharper for the lymphatic than either the myeloid or monocytic subtypes (MacMahon and Clark, 1956). Although these features have been observed in several countries, such as the United States (MacMahon and Clark, 1956) England and Wales, New Zealand and Denmark (Court Brown et al., 1964; Burnet, 1958), the myeloid subtype appears to predominate in Norway (Bjelke, 1963), even in early childhood (Figure 5.2). It has also been suggested that acute lymphatic leukaemia is less common in certain African countries (Amsel and Nambesi, 1974). Although these different

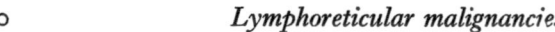

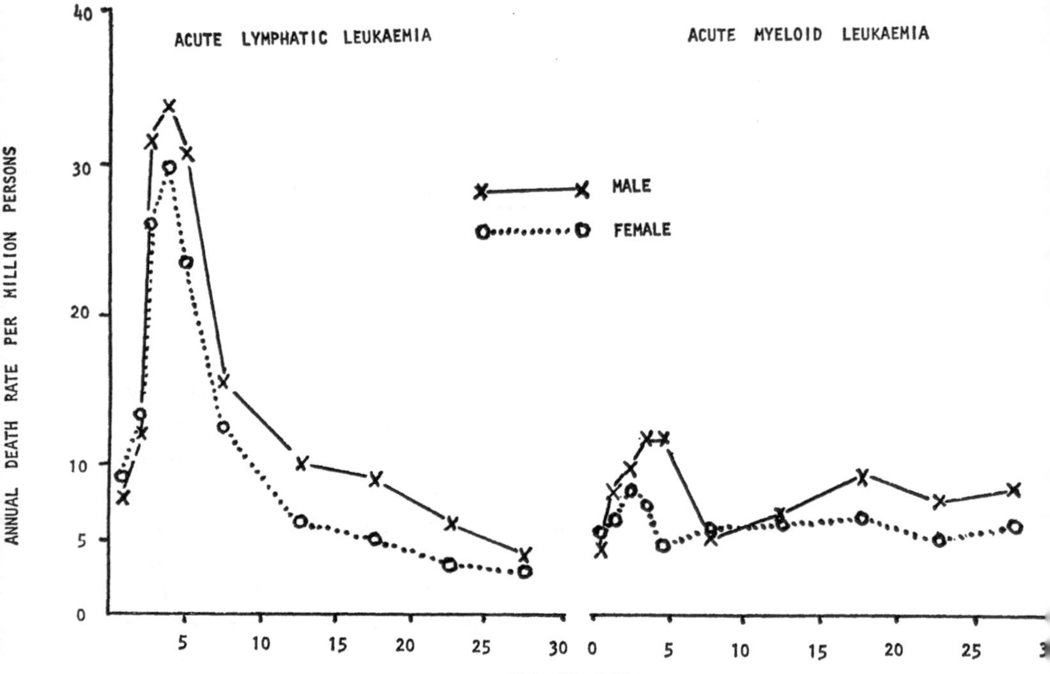

ANNUAL DEATH RATE PER MILLION PERSONS

ACUTE LYMPHATIC LEUKAEMIA

ACUTE MYELOID LEUKAEMIA

X————X MALE

O·········O FEMALE

AGE IN YEARS

Figure 5.1 Estimated age-specific death rates from acute lymphatic leukaemia and acute myeloid leukaemia under the age of 30 years by sex in England and Wales, 1945–59. (From Court Brown, W. and Doll, R. (1961), by courtesy of *Brit. Med. J.*)

patterns might be attributable in part to a variability in diagnostic criteria, they are also compatible with the possibility that different environmental factors might be important for each variety of acute leukaemia. Admittedly other factors might be invoked to explain the low incidence of acute lymphatic leukaemia in certain parts of Africa, but if these factors are related solely to genetic differences between white and non-white children, a similar pattern might be expected for non-white children in the other countries, such as the United States. Although childhood leukaemia mortality rates have generally been lower for non-whites in the United States (Table 5.1), Fraumeni and Miller (1967a) found an age peak at 3–4 years for non-whites similar to that previously found in whites. It will be of great importance to determine whether this age peak persists for non-whites in the future and if their rates eventually approximate those for whites. This possibility is not as remote as it may appear, since in England, the 3 and 4 year age peak was first apparent after 1920, but in the United States, only

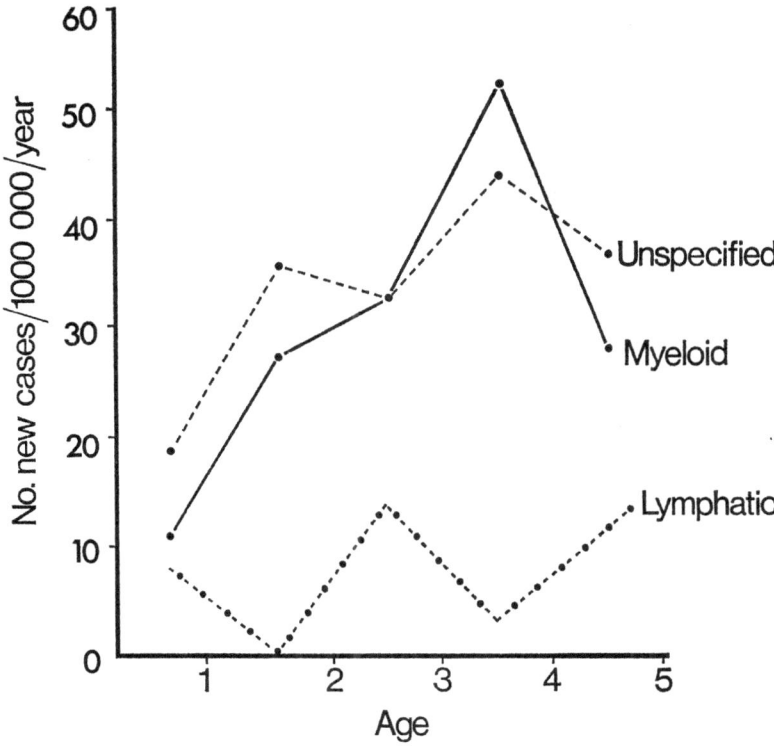

Figure 5.2 Age–specific incidence of acute leukaemia in young persons by cytological type during 1953–58 in Norway. (From Bjelke, E. (1964), by courtesy of *Cancer*)

after 1940 (Court Brown and Doll, 1961; Burnet, 1958). Furthermore, these age peaks in both countries have become more pronounced with time.

There is additional evidence suggesting that the lymphatic variety might differ from the myelogenous, undifferentiated and monocytic subtypes of acute childhood leukaemia. Fraumeni *et al.* (1971) found the lymphatic subtype to be characterised by a sharp age incidence peak at 2–3 years of age, a sex ratio close to unity and long survival. The myelogenous and undifferentiated categories varied less with age, predominated among males and had a survival pattern midway between trends for the lymphatic and monocytic types. These investigators also suggested that the proportion of leukaemias diagnosed as lymphatic increased with time over the period 1947–65 while the undifferentiated category decreased. Time trends for the various subtypes could not be

Table 5.1 Comparison of the incidence of adult and childhood leukaemias on two continents by race, male and female rates combined.
(From Amsel, S. and Nabembesi, J. S. (1974), by courtesy of J. Nat. Cancer. Inst.)

	All ages			≤ 14 years		
	Metropolitan Atlanta, Georgia*		Kyadondo County	Cuyahoga County, Ohio†		Kyadondo County
	White	Black	Black	White	Black	Black
AML – – – –	1·9	1·0	0·8			
ALL – – – –	1·7	1·3	0·7	3·9	1·6	2·0
CML – – –	1·5	1·1	0·9			
CLL – – –	2·8	1·1	0·6			

* Derived from the data of McPhedran *et al.* (21). Monocytic, stem cell and other cases omitted
† AML and ALL combined

determined however, since this was a hospital based study. Another important difference is that in contrast to the other types of acute leukaemia, the risk of the lymphatic variety is increased among children of early birth order and/or older mothers (Stark and Mantel, 1969). Furthermore, different genetic disorders apparently predispose to specific types of leukaemia. Thus, ataxia-telangiectasia is associated with lymphatic leukaemia, whereas in Fanconi's aplastic anaemia there is an increased risk of monocytic leukaemia and in Bloom's syndrome, the myelogenous subtypes (Bloom *et al.*, 1966; Miller 1967; Fraumeni, 1969).

Other observations suggest that differences might be present within various age groups of certain subtypes of childhood leukaemia. In the United States (Fraumeni and Miller, 1967a) and Norway (Glattre, 1970) a decline in leukaemia mortality rates have been observed for all age groups. In England and Wales, this decline was limited to those less than 5 years of age. There is also evidence to suggest that the appearance of the classical childhood mortality peak, due to acute leukaemia in the United States, resulted from both a decline in rates for the under-2-year age group (Figure 5.3) and an increase for those 3–4 years of age (Slocumb and MacMahon, 1963). These variations in trends are insufficient to suggest that aetiologic differences exist between different age groups with the same cell type of acute childhood leukaemia. They do, however, provide an important clue with respect to the lymphatic subtype, the most common form of childhood leukaemia in several countries. The greatest epidemiologic differences exist between the lymphatic and other varieties of acute leukaemia, 0–9 years of age, and

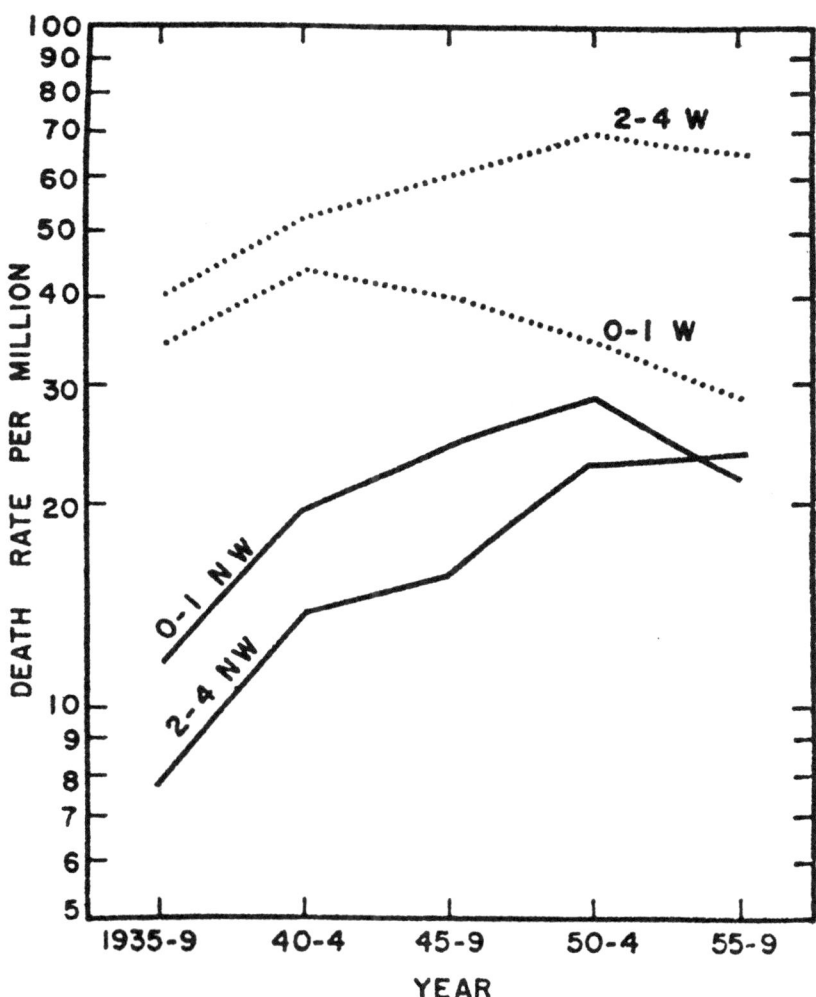

Figure 5.3 Trends in average annual death rates from leukaemia, for whites (W) and non-whites (NW) in two age groups, United States (1939–59). (From Slocumb, J. and MacMahon, B. (1963), by courtsey of *New Eng. J. Med.*)

accordingly this age group should be examined separately. Furthermore, based on different trends observed for various age groups of childhood leukaemia and the fact that an age peak occurs at 2–3 years of age (at diagnosis), it would seem most appropriate to examine the under-2-, 2–3- and 4–9-year age groups separately when factors such as seasonality are considered.

SEASONALITY IN ACUTE LYMPHATIC LEUKAEMIA OF
CHILDHOOD

The possibility that seasonal factors might affect the incidence of acute lymphatic leukaemia is an important consideration, due to the implications this might have with regard to an environmental and possibly viral aetiology for this disorder. Lee (1962; 1963) examined cases of leukaemia in patients under the age of 20 years by month of clinical onset and found an excess number during the summer, especially June. This seasonal variation was found in both male and female patients in England and Wales. Further analysis indicated that this summer peak was significant only for patients aged 5–19 years. With regard to cell types, the summer excess was noticeable in the lymphatic and unspecified varieties but not in the myeloid or monocytic. Knox (1964) also found a summer excess for cases of acute lymphatic and undifferentiated leukaemia with onsets before 15 years of age in Northumberland and Durham. In contrast Fraumeni (1963) studied leukaemia children under 16 years of age in the United States and observed an excess of cases with clinical onset during winter and spring months. Interestingly this seasonal pattern was found for the lymphatic, myeloid and monocytic subtypes but not the unspecified variety. Significance however, was limited to the acute lymphatic type. A predominance in the winter and spring months was also observed by Hayes (1961) for cases of acute leukaemia of all ages seen in a single hospital in the United States. In Norway (Bjelke, 1963) examination of cases of acute leukaemia in patients less than 20 years of age at diagnosis revealed no seasonal trend by month of diagnosis. Fraumeni *et al.* (1971) studied acute childhood leukaemia, under 15 years of age in Boston and found no significant variation in the month of clinical onset or birth for each cell type. Bailar and Gurin (1964) examined the cases of childhood leukaemia (all subtypes), 0–14 years of age, by month of birth. While no significant seasonality was observed for either sex, they did find a slight excess of births in the late summer and early fall. The results of studies on seasonality must therefore be considered to be conflicting, especially when one contrasts the patterns observed in the United States and Great Britain. While it is possible that different seasonal patterns do exist in various countries, it seems likely that some of the differences observed might be due to the variability in the approaches taken with respect to subtype and age groups. Furthermore, little attention has been given to the possibility that urban–rural differences might be present, not only in the incidence of different types of acute leukaemia, but also in their seasonal patterns. Knox (1964) found a marked difference in urban–rural rates for children with acute lymphatic and undifferentiated leukaemia aged 6–14 years at the onset of their illness. In contrast, rates for the 0–5-year age group were comparable. It must also be realised that month of onset or diagnosis may not be relevant temporal markers in acute lymphatic leukaemia of childhood. If some postnatal exposure is an essential cause of this disorder and the time interval between this event and clinical onset were variable, seasonality would not be observed. These considerations; the experimental observation that some viruses can cause a variety of tumours when injected into new-born animals (Allison, 1968), rarely if ever produce tumours in the adult (e.g. polyoma virus in mice), and the epidemiologic evidence suggesting the importance of certain prenatal exposures (e.g. radiation, viral) in childhood leukaemia (Stewart *et al.*, 1956; Stewart *et al.*, 1958), all indicate the potential importance of evaluating the lymphatic subtype by month of birth. The observation of a high concordance rate of child-hood leukaemia in monozygotic twins also suggests the potential importance of prenatal factors (MacMahon and Levy, 1964). However, for reasons already mentioned, age and urban-rural factors should be considered. Using the resources of the tumour registry of the Cancer Control Bureau, New York State Department of Health, it was possible to conduct this type of study. Months of birth for all reported cases of acute lymphatic leukaemia, occurring among residents of upstate New York, 0–9 years of age at onset of illness, were evaluated (Vianna and Polan, 1974). Cases were divided into three age groups, less than 2, 2–3 and 4–9 years of age (at onset). Cases from each age group were then further divided into two additional groups, depending upon whether they were born in urban or rural counties of upstate New York. Analysis of the 777 cases of acute lymphatic leukaemia in this manner, suggested the following seasonality in urban counties: January–April, under-2-year age group; May–October, 2–3-year age group; and July–December, 4–9-year age group. In all instances the number of cases observed was significantly greater than expected by chance. In rural counties, only the less than two year had a significant periodicity which was the same as that observed for this age group in urban regions. No significant seasonality by month of birth was observed for the 694 cases of acute unspecified leukaemia which served as a comparison group, when the same age groups and type of county (urban or rural) were examined.

These observations suggest that exposure to some environmental factor during the prenatal or natal periods might be important in the aetiology of acute childhood lymphatic leukaemia. One way of evaluating the possibility that some natal exposure might be important is to compare the rates of lymphatic leukaemia for each of the three age groups by year of birth. This was done and rank correlations of the trends of each of the three possible pairs were not statistically significant. Thus, it is most likely that the seasonality by month of birth, observed for each age group with the lymphatic subtype, is indicative of some prenatal influence. The observation that no single group of birth months predominated for all of the age groups studied suggests further that the different age groups (less than 2, 2–3, 4–9 years) might be exposed during different trimesters, but with each trimester consisting of the same specific group of months. If exposure occurred during different trimesters with no monthly specificity, this should be reflected by the absence of seasonality by month of birth. Furthermore, certain birth months should predominate for all three age groups, if exposure were during a single trimester consisting of the same specific group of months. It must be realised, however, that while the evidence presented suggests the importance of some prenatal exposure, postnatal factors might also be required for acute lymphatic leukaemia to occur. One additional observation of possible importance is that the seasonality observed was significant in urban counties for all age groups but not in rural areas. If the same leukaemogenic factors are present in both types of county, then it seems likely that they might operate with a greater degree of regularity in urban than rural counties.

POSSIBLE ASSOCIATION BETWEEN MATERNAL VIRAL INFECTION DURING PREGNANCY AND ACUTE LYMPHATIC LEUKAEMIA IN CHILDHOOD

In 1958 Stewart and Hewitt suggested that an association might exist between childhood cancer and viral infection in pregnancy. Based on the paucity of reports, this suggestion has not been given sufficient consideration until recently. In 1972 Fedrick and Alberman reported the results of a longitudinal study of close to 2000 infants born during the first week of March, 1958 to mothers who were reported to have had influenza during pregnancy. Their results suggested that the incidence of acute leukaemia in children whose mothers reported an influenza-like illness during pregnancy was significantly higher than that observed for infants of mothers who did not have this illness. These investigators also compared the prevalence of influenza in England and Wales during each winter from 1955–64 with the number of children born during the following year who subsequently died of cancer. The correlation between the number of cases of neoplasms of the lymphatic and haematopoietic tissue and the prevalence of influenza in the year preceding their birth was significant. This was also true when cases of leukaemia alone were considered. However, in a study of cohorts of children born in the Manchester region after six influenza epidemics (between 1951 and 1968), Leck and Steward (1972) found the incidence of neoplasia in this group to be no higher than that found among cohorts born in non-epidemic years during the same period. Another study in Finland (Hakulinen *et al.*, 1973), identified six influenza epidemics between 1953 and 1959 and found no association with the development of childhood leukaemia, under 10 years of age. A significant association was found between this disease and the 1957 Asian influenza epidemic, an observation which raised the possibility that there might be some relationship between maternal infection with a mutant strain of influenza and the subsequent development of childhood leukaemia. At present the evidence implicating maternal influenza and childhood leukaemia is conflicting and additional studies will be required.

There have been other studies of the possible association between various viral infections during pregnancy and childhood leukaemia. Adelstein and Donovan (1972) followed children of mothers who were reported to have varicella, mumps or rubella as a complication of pregnancy. Death certificates from this group of children between the ages of 2 and 19 years were examined and among the 270 children of mothers with chicken pox, two deaths from leukaemia were observed. In a follow-up report (Adelstein and Donovan, 1974) these investigators found no cases of childhood leukaemia among 553 mothers with influenza complicating pregnancy, 78 with Herpes zoster, 525 with mumps, 860 with rubella, 38 with measles and 173 with infectious hepatitis. In a retrospective case control–study, based on the Oxford survey of childhood cancers, Bithell *et al.* (1973) obtained histories of viral infection during pregnancy by interviewing the mothers of 9000 children who had died of cancer under the age of 16 years. The most impressive results related childhood leukaemia to maternal varicella; there were three children who died of leukaemia and had mothers with this infection as compared to mothers of children in the control group.

Although two studies suggest that maternal varicella might be associated with the childhood leukaemia, probably the lymphatic subtype, this observation must be regarded as preliminary and requiring further evaluation.

Two further comments can be made concerning the eleven identified cases of childhood leukaemia among mothers whose pregnancy was complicated by either an influenza (Fedrick and Alberman, 1972) like illness or varicella (Adelstein and Donovan, 1972; Bithell *et al.*, 1973). In ten instances the offspring developed acute lymphatic leukaemia and the age of the eleventh case (4·5 years at onset) makes it likely that she (Adelstein and Donovan, 1972) also had this subtype. The age of onset for all cases ranged from 2 to 11 years, but nine were 9 years of age or less. None of the studies were conducted in a fashion that would exclude either different leukaemia subtypes or older cases. These observations can therefore be taken as additional evidence suggesting that the 0–9-year age group of acute lymphatic leukaemia should be examined separately.

Hypothesis—*Maternal infection with varicella during the various trimesters of pregnancy might be related to the development of acute lymphatic leukaemia in different childhood age groups.*

At present, varicella must be viewed as a possible aetiologic candidate in childhood lymphatic leukaemia and evaluation of seasonality by month of birth suggests that the three age groups might be exposed during different trimesters, but with each trimester consisting of the same specific group of months (Vianna and Polan, 1974). While the evidence supporting both concepts is far from established, one can speculate that if the viral disease and leukaemic process are related, there should be some consistency in the epidemiologic characteristics of the two. In upstate New York seasonality for leukaemia was observed only in urban counties. The months of peak activity for varicella, based on case reports, extended from January through April; in urban counties this seasonality is remarkably regular whereas in rural areas a significant number of months of peak activity deviated from the prevalent monthly pattern. Significant differences in urban-rural seasonality were also observed for rubeola but not rubella or influenza.

Comparison of time trends of childhood leukaemia and varicella is another means of evaluating the possibility that the two processes might be related (Vianna and Polan, 1974). In the United States, it has been suggested that leukaemogenic factors might have been prevalent around

1940, for the 3-year age peak became evident for the first time around this time (Gilliam and Walter, 1958). Thereafter, mortality rates increased gradually to around 1950 and then levelled off (Fraumeni and Miller, 1967b). The first decline in childhood leukaemia mortality rates was observed during the period 1961–65 (Fraumeni and Miller, 1967b). In upstate New York the reported incidence for lymphatic leukaemia, 0–14 years of age, also showed a decline when yearly rates during the 1961–65 period (average incidence, 2·6/100 000 population) were compared with those from 1950–54 (average incidence, 6·7/100 000 population). Although admittedly crude, it would be reasonable to expect a likely viral candidate for this type of leukaemia to be characterised by high rates just prior to 1940, lower rates before 1950 and the lowest rates around 1961. Based on reported incidence data, obtained from the Bureau of Epidemiology, New York State Department of Health, the average of the annual incidence rates of varicella, rubella and rubeola were compared during specified periods (Table 5.2). Only varicella manifested the desired pattern.

Table 5.2 Average of the annual incidence rates of varicella, rubeola and rubella during the years 1936–40, 1946–50 and 1957–61, in upstate New York excluding New York City

| Time periods (years) | Annual incidence rates (per 100 000 population) | | |
	Varicella	Rubeola	Rubella
1936–40	257·8	461·0	· 26·8
1946–50	234·0	473·1	Not reported during this period
1957–61	193·4	314·4	89·3

Unfortunately this approach could not be employed for influenza since it is not a reportable disease in upstate New York. However, if a relationship exists between maternal-fetal infection with this agent and lymphatic leukaemia in childhood, then an influenza peak should be associated with increased leukaemia rates during the same year and/or the one immediately thereafter when cohort live birth rates for the latter are examined. From 1950 through 1960, three influenza peaks were identified. No significant difference between cohort rates of lymphatic leukaemia, 0–9 years of age, was observed when rates for the year preceding an influenza peak were compared either to those during or one year after the epidemic (Vianna and Polan, 1974).

Analyses of urban–rural differences and crude trends suggest (as do the previously described cohort and case–control studies) that varicella appears to be the most likely candidate of the viral diseases considered. The question now becomes which group of consecutive prenatal months during a calendar year do the less than 2-, 2–3- and 4–9-year age groups of childhood lymphatic leukaemia have in common which is consistent both with the different seasonality (by month of birth) observed for each age and the months of peak activity for varicella, January through April. The appropriate trimester, that is the period of likely (although hypothetical) exposure for each age group is indicated in Table 5.3. Monthly rates for the period 1950–61 were computed for cases of acute lymphatic leukaemia placed in the months of their appropriate trimester and for varicella. Rank correlation of the twelve-monthly rates for each disorder was statistically significant for all age groups in urban counties and none in rural counties. Proceeding one step further, reported incidence trends for varicella in the four largest urban counties of upstate New York were compared with lymphatic leukaemia rates, obtained by placing cases from each age group in the year of their appropriate trimester during the period 1950–61. When the magnitude and direction of the 10-year changes for both processes were evaluated, the rank correlation was statistically significant (Vianna and Polan, 1974). All of the observations mentioned in this section must be considered as preliminary but they are consistent with the possibility that maternal–fetal infection with varicella might be associated with the subsequent development of childhood lymphatic leukaemia. At present this must be considered to be a most promising hypothesis with regard to the aetiology of this disorder.

Table 5.3 Proposed trimester of prenatal exposure to varicella for the under-2, 2–3- and 4–9-year age groups of acute lymphatic leukaemia

Age groups of acute lymphatic leukaemia (age at onset)	Seasonality by month of birth (urban counties)	Appropriate trimester*
less than 2	January–April	Third
2–3	May–October	Second
4–9	July–December	First

* Based on the January–April seasonality for varicella.

OTHER CONSIDERATIONS

An important question at this juncture is whether varicella possesses any additional characteristics which make it a likely candidate in acute lymphatic leukaemia of childhood? It is well-established that this virus is lymphotactic, even to the extent that it can induce lymphocytic leukaemoid reactions simulating acute leukaemia (Goldman, 1930). This is a characteristic it shares with other herpes viruses such as the Epstein–Barr virus, and it will be quite interesting to determine whether varicella has any specific lymphocyte trophism as EBV does (Pattengale *et al.*, 1974). Placental transmission probably occurs (Overall and Glasglow, 1970) and of equal importance varicella can induce chromosomal breakage (Aula, 1963). These factors might be responsible in part for the fourfold excess of leukaemia that occurs among sibs of leukaemic children (Miller, 1963). Other important features of varicella include its capacity for prolonged latent periods (Chang, 1971) and its close relationship with herpes zoster. Both disorders are different manifestations of infection with the same viral agent. Varicella is primarily a disease of childhood (Figure 5.4) and is highly contagious, whereas herpes zoster occurs mainly in adults and the majority of patients give a previous history of varicella. These observations are indicative of the prolonged latent period this agent is capable of and it seems possible that zoster might occur when immunity from chickenpox has waned (Sieler, 1949). Additional important features of zoster include: a seasonality similar to that for varicella (Sieler, 1949), although both disorders can occur in all seasons (Simons, 1951); an attack is usually precipitated by some stressful situation, including pregnancy, (Sieler, 1949) and second attacks rarely occur. While this might explain why more than one fetus of an infected mother rarely develops clinical disease, it is important to realise that fetal infection *in utero* may occur despite maternal immunity. Indeed cases of varicella have been reported in infants of mothers not clinically ill (Pridham, 1913) but viremic. These facts could provide an explanation for the increased risk of acute lymphatic leukaemia among children of early birth order and/or older mothers (Stark and Mantel, 1969). These factors, which operate independently, have never been understood. The frequency curve for herpes zoster is clearly consistent with the likelihood that older pregnant females have an increased risk of developing this disorder and possibly leukaemia in the offspring. Quite separately, if pregnancy can be a precipitating factor for herpes zoster and one attack confers some degree of immunity it would be reasonable to expect this clinical disorder to complicate first pregnancies with the greatest frequency. Furthermore, the capacity of this virus to persist latently over prolonged periods, even in the immunised host, might explain the fourfold excess of leukaemia

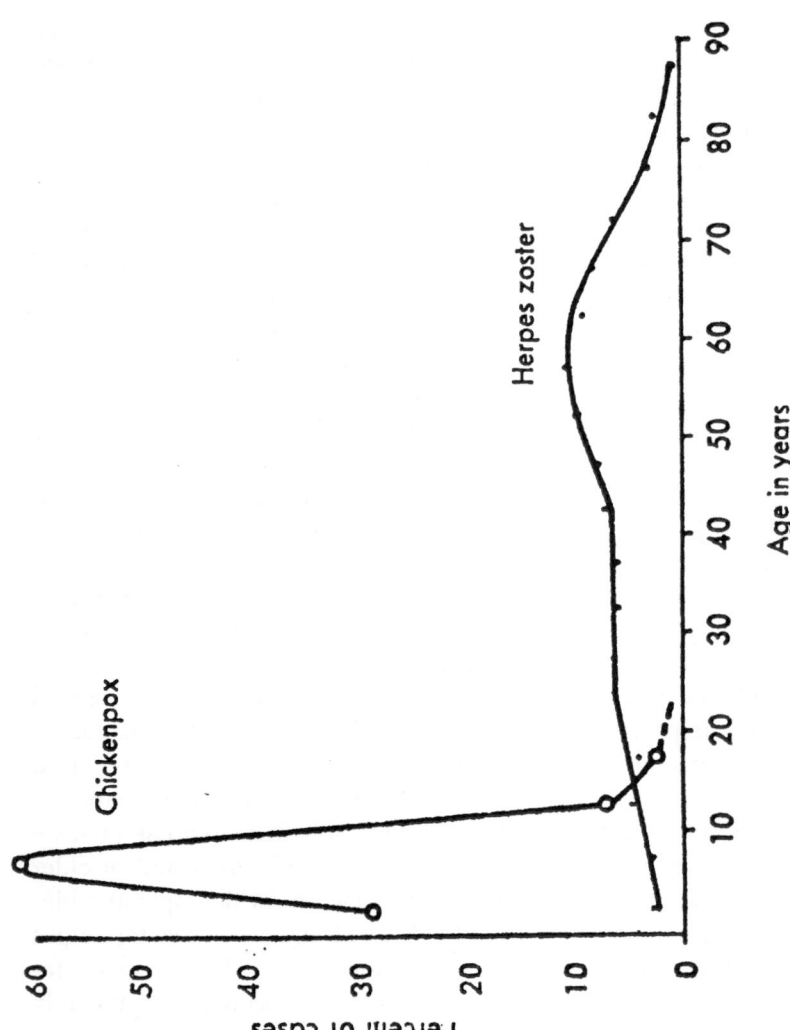

Figure 5.4 Relative frequency of varicella and herpes zoster infections at various ages. (From Karzon, D. T. (1968), by courtesy of *McGraw Hill Inc.*)

observed among the sibs of leukaemic children (Miller, 1963). It would appear that, although the association with childhood leukaemia is not firmly established, the varicella–zoster model proposed might explain many of the epidemiologic characteristics of this neoplastic disorder. What is more important to realise at this time is that, if these obervations are relevant biologically to lymphatic leukaemia in childhood, studies which identify retrospectively clinical cases of varicella zoster complicating pregnancy might relate only to the tip of the iceberg. It may well be that the majority of leukaemic cases are associated with silent maternal–fetal infection. If true, long-term prospective sero-epidemiologic studies will be required to definitively evaluate these hypotheses. This approach would also be useful in evaluating the possibility that different strains of a virus might be associated with acute lymphatic leukaemia. For example the phenomenon of antigenic drift is well-established in influenza and aberrant forms of varicella–zoster virus have been described (Nii, 1973).

References

Adelstein, A. M. and Donovan, J. W.: Malignant disease in children whose mothers had chickenpox, mumps or rubella in pregnancy. *Brit. Med. J.*, **4**:629, 1972.

Adelstein, A. M. and Donovan, J. W.: Sequelae of viral infection in pregnancy. *Brit. Med. J.*, **2**:502, 1974.

Allison, A. C.: Do viruses cause cancer in man? *Lancet*, **1**:1141, 1968.

Amsel, S. and Nabembesi, J. S.: Two-year survey of hematologic malignancies in Uganda. *J. Nat. Cancer Inst.*, **52**:1397, 1974.

Aula, P.: Chromosome breaks in leukocytes in chickenpox patients. *Hereditas*, **49**:451, 1963.

Bailar, J. C. and Gurian, J. M.: Month of birth and cancer mortality. *J. Nat. Cancer Inst.*, **33**:237, 1964.

Bithell, J. F., Draper, G. J. and Borbach, P. D.: Association between malignant disease in children and maternal virus infections. *Brit. Med. J.*, **1**:706, 1973.

Bjelke, E.: Leukaemia in children and young adults in Norway. *Cancer*, **17**:248, 1963.

Bloom, G. E., Warner, S., Gerald, P. S. *et al.*: Chromosome abnormalities in constitutional aplastic anemia. *New Eng. J. Med.*, **274**:8, 1966.

Burnet, M.: Leukaemia as a problem in preventive medicine. *New Eng. J. Med.*, **259**: 423, 1958.

Chang, T. W.: Recurrent viral infection (reinfection). *New Eng. J. Med.*, **284**:765, 1971.

Court Brown, W. M. and Doll, R.: Leukemia in childhood and young adult life: trends in mortality in relation to etiology. *Brit. Med. J.*, **1**:981, 1961.

Court Brown, W. M., Doll, R. and Hill, I. D.: Leukaemia in Britain and Scandinavia. *Pathol. Microbiol.*, **27**:644, 1964.

Epstein, M. A.: Possible role of viruses in human cancer. *Lancet*, **1**:1344, 1971.

Fedrick, J. and Alberman, E. D.: Reported influenza in pregnancy and subsequent cancer in the child. *Brit. Med. J.*, **2**:485, 1972.

Fraumeni, J. F.: Seasonal variation in leukemia incidence. *Brit. Med. J.*, **2**:12, 1963.

Fraumeni, J. F.: Clinical epidemiology of leukemia. *Seminars Haematol.*, **6**:250, 1969.

Fraumeni, J. F. and Miller, R. W.: Epidemiology of human leukemia: recent observations. *J. Nat. Cancer Inst.*, **38**:593, 1967a.

Fraumeni, J. F. and Miller, R. W.: Leukemia mortality: downturn in the United States. *Science*, **155**:1126, 1967b.

Fraumeni, J. F., Manning, M. D. and Mitus, W. J.: Acute childhood leukemia: epidemiologic study by cell type of 1,263 cases at Children's Cancer Research Foundation in Boston, 1947–1965. *J. Nat. Cancer Inst.*, **46**:461, 1971.

Gilliam, A. G. and Walter, W. A.: Trends of mortality from leukemia in the United States, 1921–1955. *Public Health Rep.*, **73**:773, 1958.

Glattre, E.: Leukemia mortality in Norway. *Lancet*, **1**:526, 1970.

Goldman, D.: Chickenpox with a blood picture simulating that in leukemia. *Amer. J. Dis. Child.*, **40**:1282, 1930.

Gross, L.: *Oncogenic Viruses*, 140–183 (Oxford: Pergamon, 1961).

Hakulinen, T., Hovi, L., Karkinen-Jaaskelaninen, M., Penttinen, K. *et al.*: Association between influenza during pregnancy and childhood leukemia. *Brit. Med. J.*, **4**:265, 1973.

Hayes, D. M.: Seasonal incidence of acute leukemia. *Cancer*, **14**:1301, 1961.

Karzon, D. T.: Chickenpox (varicella) and Herpes Zoster. In: *The Biologic Basis of Pediatric Practice*, 639 (R. E. Cooke, editor) (McGraw Hill Inc.).

Knox, G.: Epidemiology of childhood leukemia in Northumberland and Durham. *Brit. J. Prev. Soc. Med.*, **18**:17, 1964.

Leck, J. and Steward, J. K.: Incidence of neoplasms in children born after influenza epidemics. *Brit. Med. J.*, **4**:631, 1972.

Lee, J. A. H.: Seasonal variation in clinical onset of leukemia in young people. *Brit. Med. J.*, **1**:1737, 1962.

Lee, J. A. H.: Seasonal variation in leukemia incidence. *Brit. Med. J.*, **2**:623, 1963.

MacMahon, B. and Clark, D.: Incidence of common forms of human leukemia. *Blood*, **11**:871, 1956.

MacMahon, B. and Levy, A.: Prenatal origin of childhood leukemia. *New Eng. J. Med.*, **270**:1082, 1964.

Miller, R. W.: Down's syndrome (Mongolism), other congenital malformations and cancers among sibs of leukemic children. *New Eng. J. Med.*, **268**:393, 1963.

Miller, R. W.: Persons with exceptionally high risk of leukemia: recent observations. *Cancer Res.*, **27**:2420, 1967.

Nii, S.: Aberrant forms of varicella-zoster virus. *Biken Journal*, **16**:173, 1973.

Overall, J. C. and Glasglow, L. A.: Virus infections of the fetus and newborn infant. *J. Pediat.*, **77**:315, 1970.

Pattengale, P. K., Smith, R. W. and Gerber, P.: B-cell characteristics of human peripheral and cord blood lymphocytes transformed by Epstein–Barr virus. *J. Nat. Cancer Inst.*, **52**:1081, 1974.

Pridham, F. C.: Chickenpox during intrauterine life. *Brit. Med. J.*, **1**:1054, 1913.

Sieler, H. E.: A study of herpes zoster, particularly its relationship to chickenpox. *J. Hygiene*, **47**:253, 1949.

Simons, R. D. G.: Some climatological and other particulars on herpes zoster from the Northern and Southern hemispheres. *Dermatologica*, (**No. 2**), **103**: 109, 1951.

Slocumb, J. C. and MacMahon, B.: Changes in mortality rates from leukemia in the first five years of life. *New Eng. J. Med.*, **268**:922, 1963.

Stark, C. R. and Mantel, N.: Maternal age and birth-order effects in childhood leukemia: age of child and type of leukemia. *J. Nat. Cancer Inst.*, **42**:857. 1969.

Stewart, A., Webb, J., Giles, D. and Hewitt, D.: Malignant disease in childhood and diagnostic irradiation *in utero*. *Lancet*, **2**:447, 1956.

Stewart, A., Webb, J. and Hewitt, D.: A survey of childhood malignancies. *Brit. Med. J.*, **1**:1495, 1958.

Vianna, N. J. and Polan, A.: Childhood lymphatic leukemia: seasonality and possible association with congenital varicella (in press).

CHAPTER 6

Childhood lymphomas

If environmental factors are important in the aetiology of the major lymphomas, then much is to be gained from evaluating this group of disorders in children. There are several reasons for this. In most of the world, children are exposed to less than adults; their environment is relatively confined and therefore more definable, quantitatively and qualitatively. It should also be appreciated that there is an adult counterpart to Hodgkin's disease, lymphosarcoma and reticulum cell sarcoma in childhood. Putting aside the question whether each of these disorders is similar aetiologically in both age groups, intensive investigation of the lymphomas in the young can provide us with some facts relevant to older age groups. The study of childhood lymphomas as a group also affords the opportunity to evaluate the possible role of chromosomal and/or inborn immunologic defects as predisposing factors. This approach has already produced many dividends and as our ability to detect more subtle congenital defects improves, additional information of great importance will undoubtedly be gained. We know of the association between maternal radiation (Stewart and Kneale, 1970), mongolism, Kleinfelter's syndrome and various autosomal recessive defects (Fraumeni, 1969) and certain types of leukaemia. We have also learned that certain immunologic deficiencies (the Wiskott–Aldrich syndrome, Chediak–Higashi syndrome, ataxia-telangiectasia) predispose to the lymphomas (Miller, 1968). We must now ask what other disorders, in addition to those which are readily apparent clinically, might increase ones risk of developing a lymphoreticular malignancy? Another reason for studying this group separately is that they have certain distinctive epidemiologic features which set them apart both from other malignant diseases in the young and from similar disorders in the old. But perhaps the most important reason for devoting all our efforts to this group of diseases is that they are a major cause of morbidity and mortality in children, and as such they must be viewed as tragic disorders. Although major advances have been made in therapy, our goal must still be to prevent these disorders. This can be accomplished only by identifying predisposing factors and interrupting the chain of events which ultimately leads to the development of these disorders. As a starting point, however, one must look for differences in lymphoma patterns.

INCIDENCE PATTERNS OF THE COMMON CHILDHOOD LYMPHOMAS

In contrast to the Burkitt's lymphoma,, a climatically dependent lymphoreticular disorder with a relatively localised geographic distribution, the other lymphomas of childhood are widespread. In the United States (Grundy *et al.*, 1973) lymphosarcoma is the most common lymphoma in the young. This also appears to be true in France (Lemerle, 1973) and other western countries. However, in none of these areas does this tumour account for the majority of childhood neoplasms, as is the case with the Burkitt lymphoma in sections of East Africa (O'Conor and Davies, 1960). The dominant position of childhood Hodgkin's disease in South American countries has been referred to in Chapter 2 and this apparently holds true for Egypt (El-Gazayerli *et al.*, 1964) and several regions of India. For example, in West Bombay (Paymaster, 1964) and Vellore (Singh and Scudder, 1965). Hodgkin's disease accounts for a greater percentage of the childhood tumours than all other lymphomas combined. In contrast, Stewart (1964) found the other lymphomas to be about twice as common as Hodgkin's disease in Manchester, England. Indeed in this region Hodgkin's disease is the third commonest of the non-leukaemic reticuloendothelial tumours, behind lymphosarcoma and histiocytosis X (Marsden and Steward, 1968). The frequency with which these different patterns have been observed in several studies, makes it unlikely that these variations are due solely to differences in diagnostic criteria. The differences and relative importance of certain childhood lymphomas in African and Western European countries do appear to be real and the reasons behind them are undoubtedly complex. It has been stressed (Chapter 3) that the Burkitt's lymphoma is not a disease of African children but rather one of children in Africa. This and the climatic features associated with this tumour suggest the importance of environmental factors. Yet if one surveys various South American regions with virtually identical climates for this disorder, it is quite rare. Why should there be a high frequency of Hodgkin's disease in certain South American and other countries? If this is attributable solely to socio-economic development, why doesn't this disease assume a similar dominant position in Africa? It seems clear that while many of the variations in certain types of childhood lymphomas might be due to specific environmental differences, host factors must also play an important role in the development and histologic manifestations of these disorders.

If the international distribution of the childhood lymphomas is diverse, so too are the age incidence patterns for the various types within a country. In Manchester, England, lymphosarcoma affects children of all ages (Marsden and Steward, 1968), and it may have a peak in incidence, between the ages of 2 and 5 years, similar to that seen in acute leukaemia of the lymphatic type. In contrast, most cases of childhood Hodgkin's disease occur between the sixth and eighth year of life in this region. Reticulum cell sarcoma may be histologically indistinguishable from lymphosarcoma on occasion and these two disorders have been grouped together in several studies. In these hospital surveys where they have been separated (Table 6.1), it seems clear that reticulum cell sarcoma rarely occurs in children under 14 years of age. The different patterns for Hodgkin's disease, lymphosarcoma and reticulum cell sarcoma become most obvious, however, when the age–specific rates for these disorders are compared. In the United States there are few deaths from Hodgkin's disease under the age of 5 years (Miller, 1966), but between the ages of 5 and 12 years, there occurs a gradual increase in mortality rates (Figure 6.1). In contrast lymphosarcoma mortality rates rise rapidly between the ages of 0–4 years, plateau from the age of 5 years throughout most of childhood (Figure 6.2), and then decline. The mortality pattern for childhood reticulum cell sarcoma is characterised by a very gradual increase with advancing age (Grundy *et al.*, 1973). As would be expected, incidence and mortality patterns for each disorder closely parallel one another. It would seem then that each of the three lymphomas are characterised by adult peaks (Chapters 2 and 3), but only Hodgkin's disease and lymphosarcoma have either early adult or childhood peaks. It will be important to determine whether the level of urbanisation in a country has the same effect on lymphosarcoma age incidence patterns as it does on Hodgkin's disease (Chapter 2). Another important difference is that Grundy *et al.* (1973) found that from 1950 to 1969, lymphosarcoma trends decreased, whereas reticulum cell sarcoma increased.

Each of the non-Hodgkin's lymphomas in childhood have a definite male preponderance, and in this respect are similar to Hodgkin's disease. As indicated in Figure 6.1, the sex ratio in children with this disorder,

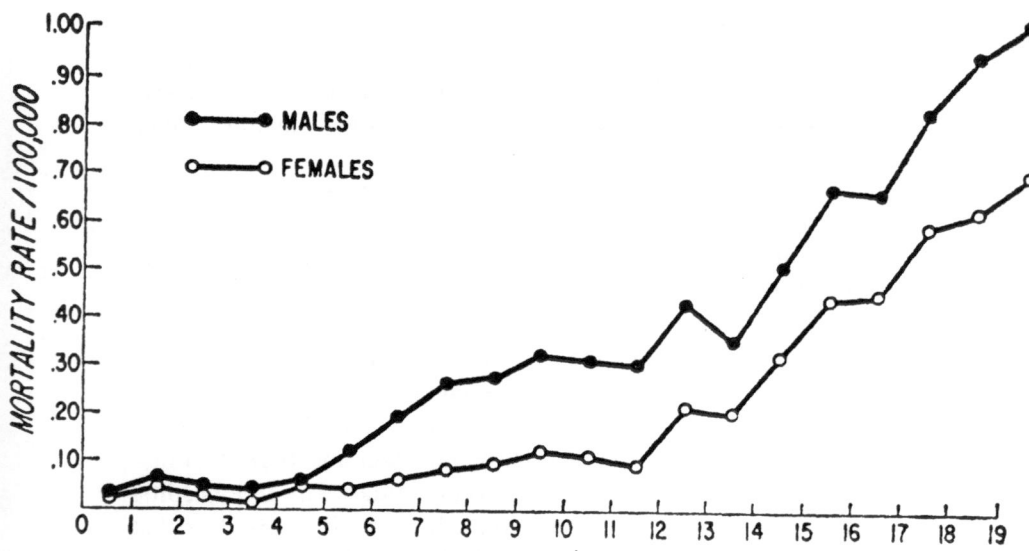

Figure 6.1 Mortality from Hodgkin's disease among US white children by single year of age and sex from 1950 to 1959. (From Miller, R. (1966), by courtesy of *J.A.M.A.*)

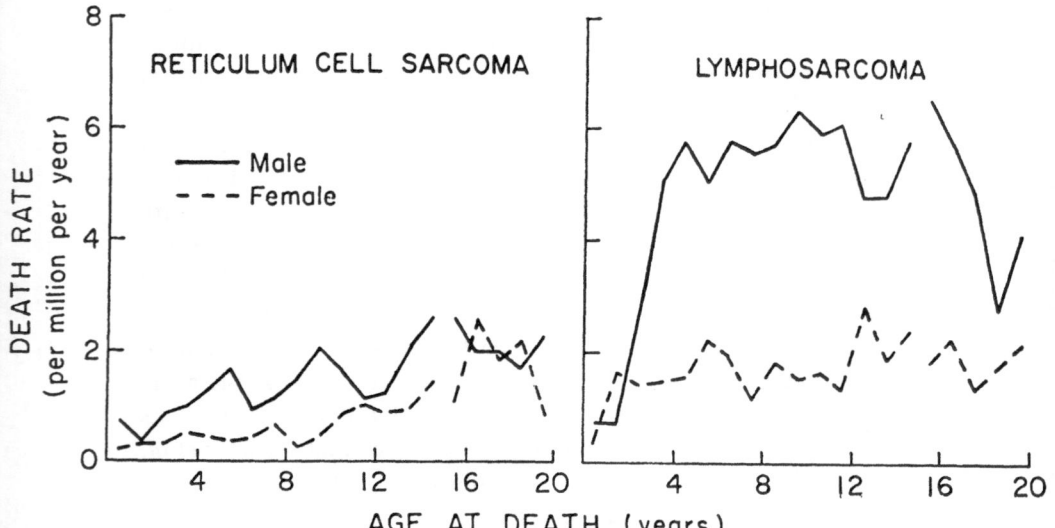

Figure 6.2 Mortality from reticulum cell sarcoma and lymphosarcoma by sex and age at death, US white children. 1960–67 (0–14 years) and 1965–67 (15–19 years). (From Grundy, G. W. (1973) by courtesy of *J. Nat. Cancer Inst.*)

Table 6.1 Comparison of the distribution of childhood lymphosarcoma and reticulum-cell sarcoma from surveys in different countries

	Lymphosarcoma (No. cases)	Reticulum-cell sarcoma (No. cases)	Total
United States (Dargeon, 1961)	44	31	75
France (Lemerle et al., 1973)	112	60	172
Egypt (El-Gazayerli et al., 1964)	6	0	6

5 to 11 years of age is about three and decreases somewhat thereafter (Miller, 1966). The number of cases occurring in the 0–4-year age group is too small to make any definitive statement about sex ratio (e.g. Miller (1966) found only twenty-two deaths due to this disease in the under-5-year age group in the United States from 1960 through 1964). Sex ratios for childhood (under 15 years of age) lymphosarcoma and reticulum cell sarcoma are 2·7:1 and 1·6:1 respectively (Grundy et al., 1973) in the United States. It is interesting that prior to 4 years of age, the sex ratio for lymphosarcoma approximates unity. This observation might have important implications with respect to leukaemic transformation in this disorder, since a characteristic feature of childhood lymphatic leukaemia is a similar incidence for both sexes.

There are other important differences which serve to separate the three major childhood lymphomas. The most common site of initial clinical presentation in Hodgkin's disease is the cervical nodes. In contrast the initial clinical site in both lymphosarcoma and reticulum cell sarcoma varies greatly (Marsden and Steward, 1968). Not infrequently these two disorders are initially localised in a non-lymphatic organ, but this is more common in reticulum cell sarcoma (Lemerle et al., 1973). Mediastinal and cervical node involvement is common in lymphosarcoma whereas bone involvement is more characteristic in reticulum cell sarcoma (Grundy et al., 1973). The vast majority of ileocecal lymphomas in childhood are of the lymphosarcoma type. Both of the non-Hodgkin's lymphomas are more rapidly progressive than Hodgkin's disease (Marsden and Steward, 1968).

The differences in incidence patterns, changes in sex ratio, initial site of presentation and progression for each of these childhood disorders, are indicative of a heterogeneity which must be considered in any aetiologic hypothesis. Further investigation of the similarities and differences in the childhood lymphomas is clearly required, especially for the non-Hodgkin's group. We know very little about the possible influence of socio-economic, urban–rural and seasonal factors in these disorders. Furthermore, there have been no systematic familial studies and we have virtually no knowledge concerning relationship patterns, sex, age and time intervals between diagnoses and the possible association between lymphoreticular disorders of different histologic types.

The student of lymphoreticular diseases must also take into account the many differences that exist between the childhood and adult age groups for each type of disorder. We have already seen the heterogeneity within Hodgkin's disease (Chapter 2). While the risk of developing lymphosarcoma and reticulum cell sarcoma increases throughout life for the most part, it must be realised that there is a peak incidence in primary gastrointestinal tract lymphoma between the ages of 5 and 8 years (Jenkin and Sonley, 1969). The sex ratio in children with each of these disorders is greater than that in the adult. Compared with the non-Hodgkin's lymphomas in adults, abdominal or mediastinal involvement is more common in childhood (Jenkin, 1974). Furthermore, these disorders are more rapidly fatal in children than adults (Rosenberg *et al.*, 1961). As is true for Hodgkin's disease, the significance of these differences is not known. Accordingly we are obliged at present to consider each age group separately. This would appear to be particularly true with regard to lymphosarcoma, which together with Hodgkin's disease and acute lymphatic leukaemia, represents another disease with a bimodal incidence curve.

LEUKAEMIA CONVERSION IN CHILDHOOD LYMPHOMAS

One of the most intriguing aspects of certain childhood lymphomas is the phenomenon of leukaemic transformation, It is important to realise one major limitation at the start: the use of therapy directed against the underlying lymphoma, denies us the opportunity to evaluate the natural history of this occurrence. But there have been several reports dealing with this problem so that we can consider certain specific questions. When compared to lymphosarcoma and reticulum cell sarcoma, Hodgkin's disease rarely terminates in acute leukaemia. Although all types of leukaemia have been associated with Hodgkin's disease, the most common is the acute non-lymphocytic variety (Burns *et al.*, 1971; Ezdini *et al.*, 1969; Gill and McCall, 1943; Johnson *et al.*, 1966;

Newman *et al.*, 1970; Scherer *et al.*, 1964). Among 1500 patients with Hodgkin's disease, three developed myelomonocytic leukaemia (Newman *et al.*, 1970). In another study, England and King (1970) found only three patients with granulocytic leukaemia among 7536 cases of Hodgkin's disease. A recent comprehensive review of this subject (Sahakian *et al.*, 1974) suggested that the incidence of acute leukaemia in Hodgkin's disease might be increasing and this might be due to aggressive treatment with radiation and drugs. If true, the occurrence of acute leukaemia should be viewed as a superimposition of a second malignancy and not a leukaemic transformation of the underlying disease. Until proven otherwise, this must be considered the most plausible hypothesis since it is most consistent with the facts that: there is an increased incidence of non-lymphatic leukaemia in patients treated with irradiation for ankylosing spondylitis (Court Brown and Doll, 1957; Van Swaay, 1955) and all patients reported in the literature with Hodgkin's disease and acute leukaemia were treated with radiation (Sahakian *et al* , 1974), albeit in different doses.

Turning to the non-Hodgkin's lymphomas, the syndrome of leukaemic conversion first described as leucosarcoma by Sternberg (1905), occurs with a much greater frequency in children than adults (Rosenberg *et al.*, 1958), and in lymphosarcoma than reticulum cell sarcoma (Gendelman *et al.*, 1969). Rosenberg and his colleagues (1961) found that leukaemic transitions occurred most commonly in children with small cell lymphosarcoma (12·6 per cent) and giant follicular lymphosarcoma (8·6 per cent). Only 2·4 per cent of reticulum cell sarcoma cases showed complete transformation. In the majority of instances the leukaemia is lymphatic in type, but occasionally it can be stem cell.

What else can be said to further categorise leukaemic transformation? In a study of childhood lymphosarcoma at Memorial Hospital, New York, Dargeon (1961) reported twenty-one cases of children (sixteen males, five females) whose primary diagnosis was lymphosarcoma, but who subsequently developed leukaemia. Of interest are the facts that all of these patients were 10 years of age or younger and in all but one instance, this complication occurred less than twenty months following the initial diagnosis. Furthermore, the cervical and mediastinal regions were the most common initial clinical sites in this group. Another study (Sullivan, 1962) of twenty-nine children with non-Hodgkin's lymphomas revealed that twelve (41 per cent) underwent leukaemic transformation. Ten of the twelve patients were initially diagnosed with lymphosarcoma. Neither of the two children with reticulum cell sarcoma became leukaemic. The average age of children with this complication was slightly lower than that for those without leukaemia (7·4 years *vs.* 8·5 years), and neither sex predominated. Leukaemic transformation did not appear to depend on whether the disease was localised or not. Splenomegaly was three times as frequent in the leukaemic group than among those without this complication and the duration of the disease at the time of conversion ranged from ten to sixty weeks (average twenty-eight weeks). Interestingly, Rosenberg *et al.* (1961) found that 75 per cent of lymphosarcoma patients with leukaemic changes had splenomegaly as opposed to 29·3 per cent for those without this transition. Lemerle *et al.* 1973 found that among 172 children aged 7 months to 14 years, 17 per cent with lymposarcoma and 11 per cent with reticulum cell sarcoma developed leukaemia. Bone marrow involvement was as frequent in initially localised disease and in advanced stages. Others have observed that leukaemic conversion is characterised by a more rapid course with neurologic complications similar to those seen in acute lymphatic leukaemia (Gendelman *et al.*, 1969). Similarities in initial symptoms, physical findings, bone marrow and peripheral blood picture and clinical course (Schwartz *et al.*, 1965) all suggest that some association between lymphosarcoma and lymphatic leukaemia might exist, especially in childhood (Fitzpatrick *et al.*, 1974). A major limitation in the above studies is that they all are based on reports from single hospitals. However, due to the consistency in certain observations, a specific pattern becomes apparent. Leukaemic transformation occurs most frequently in lymphosarcoma, especially in male children, 10 years of age or less. The occurrence of this phenomenon does not appear to be dependent on whether the underlying lymphoma is localised or not. but it is possible that involvement of a particular organ, such as the spleen, is a prerequisite. The interval between initial diagnosis and conversion to a lymphatic leukaemia picture, while variable, is relatively short. This observation and the fact that transformation occurs in both localised and disseminated disease suggests that the latter phenomenon is not a terminal event. A major systematic study (Grundy *et al.*, 1973) of 2642 United States children who died of non-Hodgkin's lymphoma from 1960 through 1967 and hospital records of 900 children was conducted to further evaluate the epidemiologic features of this group of disorders. Leukaemic transformation was noted on 11 per cent of the death certificates and 25 per cent of hospital charts. This variation in conversion percentages is probably indicative of the poor quality of death certificate information. In this report, the percentage of cases that underwent leukaemic conversion declined with increasing age (34 per cent under the age of 5 years and 6 per cent for the 15–19 age group) and the sex ratio for converted cases was greater than 2:1 (male/female). Unfortunately cases with leukaemia as a complication were not subdivided by their initial type of lymphoma

In general, then, the epidemiologic patterns observed in various hospital studies and this systematic survey are similar. Lymphosarcoma and acute lymphatic leukaemia share many common features. In addition to those which have already been mentioned, these two disorders show a maximum morbidity between the third and fifth years and there may be an increased risk of leukaemia and/or lymphoma among sib pairs (Grundy *et al.*, 1973). This latter possibility requires further detailed evaluation. Although leukaemic conversion occurs in reticulum cell sarcoma and Hodgkin's disease, neither disorder has many features in common with acute lymphatic leukaemia. A major difference between this type of leukaemia and childhood lymphosarcoma, however, is the larger sex ratio in the latter disorder. While this might be due to a variability in host response to the same aetiologic agent(s), other possibilities must be considered. It should be recalled that male predominance in childhood lymphosarcoma is considerably less under 5 years of age (Figure 6.2), the age group for which leukaemic transformation is highest. Yet the male excess, characteristic of childhood lymphosarcoma, persists for the group that undergoes transformation. Furthermore, although the nasopharynx, thymus, mucosa of the gastrointestinal tract and the cervical, mediastinal, mesenteric and retroperitoneal nodes are the most common primary sites for both sexes of childhood lymphosarcoma (Dargeon, 1953), there is a striking male excess (6·1) for involvement of the gastrointestinal tract. How might these seemingly divergent observations explain the male predominance in those cases who undergo leukaemic conversion? It seems clear that most of the lymphocytes present in lymph nodes enter these organs from the circulating blood (Hall and Morris, 1965), through cuboidal epithelium-lined venules (Gowans and Morris, 1964). In mammals, including humans (Miller, 1969) these specialised venules are limited to the lymph nodes and intestinal lymphoid tissue. This suggests that the distribution of lymphocytes (circulating *vs.* those in lymphoreticular tissue) might be influenced by the type of organs involved. Some support for this possibility is gained by the observations that leukaemic conversion is not related to whether the underlying lymphoma is localised or widespread and that many cases with this complication have enlarged

8—LM * *

spleens. Since the lymphoid tissue in the intestines of humans is largely
limited to the appendix and peyers patches, involvement of these sites
might also increase the likelihood of leukaemic conversion. Interestingly
the ileocoecal region is the most common site of gastrointestinal tract
involvement (Grundy *et al.*, 1973) and as has already been noted, this
location is associated with a male excess. It seems possible then that the
male predominance in leukaemic transformation might be related to
differences in the initial anatomic transformation of the underlying
lymphoma between the sexes. Further evaluation of this possibility
is required and laparotomy studies should be most helpful in this respect.
If splenic and gastrointestinal lesions increase the frequency of transformation, how often is involvement of one site associated with disease
in the other? The thymus is another site worthy of evaluating for
differences in the frequency of involvement in males and females. This
organ can be the primary site of lymphosarcoma in children and it is
known that certain children, primarily males, have an anterior mediastinal mass (Smith *et al.*, 1973) prior to developing acute lymphatic
leukaemia. What is of great interest in this regard is the suggestion that
these mediastinal tumours and the leukaemia that develops are of
thymic origin (Smith *et al.*, 1973). Other studies have indicated that
T-cell lymphoblastic leukaemia may represent about 20 per cent of all
cases of acute lymphatic leukaemia and that thymic involvement (or a
mediastinal mass) is not a characteristic feature of this group (Catovsky
et al., 1974). This variant of acute leukaemia is however characterised
by a more aggressive clinical course (very high peripheral blast cell
counts at onset, early meningeal leukaemia and resistance to therapy)
when compared with that type of lymphatic leukaemia which has no
markers. The implications of these observations, both with regard to
lymphoblastic leukaemia and certain lymphomas in childhood, are
obvious. How many diseases or variants of the same disease are there
in acute lymphatic leukaemia (Figure 6.3)? The epidemiologic evidence
presented in Chapter 5 also suggests a heterogeneity within this disorder.
If we assume that leukaemic conversion in childhood lymphosarcoma
is a variant of acute leukaemia (or the opposite), what are the immunologic characteristics of those cases who undergo this transformation?
Is the Burkitt tumour, a distinct type of childhood lymphoma which
none the less has certain features in common with lymphosarcoma, the
B-cell counterpart of acute lymphatic leukaemia? Does some antigenic
stimulus of the reticuloendothelial system, perhaps in the form of
chronic parasitism, tend to localise this disorder in African countries?

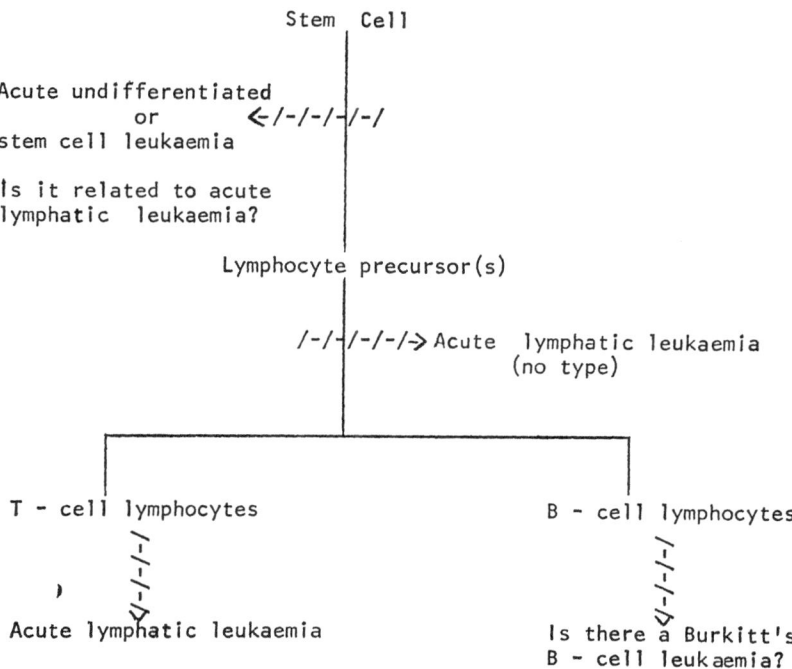

Figure 6.3 Possible immunologic variants of acute lymphatic leukaemia in childhood

If this is true, and we recall that gastrointestinal involvement is more common in American Burkitt's than in Africa, a higher frequency of leukaemic conversion might be expected in western countries, as in fact has been observed.

From what has been presented in this chapter, it should be apparent that we can no longer speak of 'all lymphomas'. When all these disorders are grouped together, there may be a lack of significant variation by single year of age throughout childhood. But when each disorder is viewed separately, rather dramatic differences are found. Hodgkin's disease and lymphosarcoma have bimodal incidence patterns; reticulum cell sarcoma does not. All three lymphomas have a male excess but sex-ratio changes vary for each. Hodgkin's disease is extremely rare under the age of 5 years whereas lymphosarcoma has a modest peak at 3–5 years. These and other differences described speak neither for nor against a different aetiology in the young and old with one disease. They do however, make clear the necessity to evaluate each age group of each lymphoma separately at present. Proceeding in this manner, we can ask specific questions such as those raised about childhood lymphosarcoma and its possible relationship with acute lymphatic leukaemia. When we have identified a likely predisposing factor for a certain lymphoreticular disease, a relevant question then becomes whether this factor is operative for each of the other disorders. To group all lymphomas together is to invite future confusion.

References

Branch, C. F.: A case of congenital lymphoblastoma, *Am. J. Path.*, 9:777, 1933.

Burns, P., Stjerholm, R. and Kellermeyer, R.: Hodgkin's disease terminating in acute lymphosarcoma cell leukemia. *Cancer*, 27:806, 1971.

Catovsky, D., Goldman, J. M., Okos, A. *et al.*: T-lymphoblastic leukemia: a distinct variety of acute leukemia. *Brit. Med. J.*, 2:643, 1974.

Chaves, E.: Hodgkin's disease in the first decade. *Cancer*, 31:925, 1973.

Court Brown, W. M. and Doll, R.; Leukemia and aplastic anemia in patients irradiated for ankylosing spondylitis. *Med. Res. Council, Spec. Rep.*, Series No. 295, 135 (London: Her Majesty's Stationery Office, 1957).

Dargeon, H. W.: Lymphosarcoma in Childhood. In: *Advances in Pediatrics*, Vol. 6, 13 (S. Z. Levine, editor) (Chicago: Year Book Publishers, 1953).

Dargeon, H. W.: Tumors of childhood. (New York: Hoeber 1960, 321).

Dargeon, H. W.: Lymphosarcoma in childhood. *Amer. J. Roentgenol. Rad. Ther. Nuc. Med.*, 85:729, 1961.

Eichler, P.: Ein fall von kogenitalem lymphosarkom des pandreas, Frankfurt. *Ztschr. J. Path.*, 36:326, 1928.

El-Gazayerli, M., Kharadly, M., Khalil, H. *et al*: Primary tumours of lymph nodes. In: *Symposium on Lymphoreticular Tumors in Africa*, 40. (F. C. Roulet, editor) (Basel, New York: S. Karger, 1964).

England, N. W. J. and King, F. M.: Relationship between Hodgkin's disease and leukemia. *International Congress of Hematology, Munich*, vol. 13, 1970, 193.

Ezdini, E. Z., Sokal, J. E. and Aungst, C. W.: Myeloid leukemia in Hodgkin's disease. *Ann. Int. Med.*, 71:1097, 1969.

Fitzpatrick, J., Lieberman, N. and Sinks, L. F.: Staging of acute leukemia and the relationship to central nervous system involvement. *Cancer*, 33:1376, 1974.

Fraumeni, J. F.: Clinical epidemiology of leukemia. *Semin. Hematol.* 6:250, 1969.

Gendelman, S., Rizzo, F. and Mones, R. J.; Central nervous system complications of leukemia conversion of the lymphomas. *Cancer*, 24:679, 1969.

Gill, W. and McCall, A. J.: Lymphadenoma and leukemia. *Brit. Med. J.*, 1:284, 1943.

Gowans, J. L. and Morris B.: The route of re-circulation of lymphocytes in the rat. *Proc. Roy. Soc. Biol.*, 195:275, 1964.

Grundy, G. W., Creagan, E. T. and Fraumeni, J. F.: Non-Hodgkin's lymphomas in childhood: epidemiologic features. *J. Nat. Cancer Inst.*, 51:767, 1973.

Hall, J. G. and Morris, B.: The origin of the cells in the efferent lymph from a single node. *J. Exp. Med.*, 121:901, 1965.

Jenkin, R. D. T. and Sonley, M. J.: *The Management of Malignant Lymphoma in Childhood*, 305 (Chicago: Year Medical Book 1969).

Jenkin, R. D. T.: The management of malignant lymphomas in childhood. In: *Modern Radiotherapy and Oncology*, 342 (T. J. Deeley, editor)(Great Britain: Butterworths 1974).

Johnson, F. D., Jacobs, E. M. and Wood, D. A.; Hodgkin's disease terminating in chronic myeloid leukemia. *Calif. Med.*, **104**:479, 1966.

Lemerle, M., Gerard-Marchant, R., Sarrazin, D. *et al.*: Lymphosarcoma and reticulum cell sarcoma in children. *Cancer*, **32**:1499, 1973.

Marsden, H. B. and Steward, J. K.: Non-leukemic tumors and leucosarcomas. In: *Tumors in Children*, 63 (Berlin, Heidelberg, New York: Springer-Verlag, 1968).

Maxwell, G. M.: Twelve cases of lymphoblastoma in children. *Arch Dis. Child.*, **29**:155. 1954.

Miller, J. J.: Studies of the phylogeny and ontogeny of the specialized lymphatic tissue venules. *Lab. Invest.*, **21**:484, 1969.

Miller, R. W.: Mortality in childhood Hodgkin's disease. *J.A.M.A.*, **198**:1216, 1966.

Miller, R. W.: Relation between cancer and congenital defects: an epidemilogic evaluation. *J. Nat. Cancer Inst.*, **40**:1079, 1968.

Murphy, M. L.: Leukemia in children. *Pediat, Clin, N. Amer.*, **6**:611, 1959.

Newman, D. R., Maldonado, J. E., Harrison, E. G. *et al.*: Myelomonocytic leukemia in Hodgkin's disease. *Cancer*, **25**:128, 1970.

O'Conor, G. T. and Davies, J. N. P.: Malignant tumors in African children. *J. Pediat.*, **56**:526, 1960.

Paymaster, J. C.: The pediatric and the geriatric aspects of cancer. *J. Indian Med. Assoc.*, **39**:163, 1964.

Rogatz, J. L.: Pleomorphous cell lymphosarcoma of thymus. *J. Pediat.*, **14**:618, 1939.

Rosenberg, S. A., Diamond, H. D., Dargeon, H. W. *et al.*: Lymphosarcoma in childhood. *New Eng. J. Med.*, **259**:505, 1958.

Rosenberg, S. A., Diamond, H. D., Jaslowitz, B. *et al.*: Lymphosarcoma: a review of 1269 cases. *Medicine*, **40**:31, 1961.

Sahakian, G. J., Al-Mondhiry, H., Lacher, M. J. *et al.*: Acute leukemia in Hodgkin's disease. *Cancer*, **33**:1369, 1974.

Scheerer, P., Pierre, R., Schwartz, D. *et al.*: Reed-Sternberg cell leukemia and lactic acidosis. *New Eng. J. Med.*, **270**:274, 1964.

Schnitzer, B., Nishiyama, R. H., Heidelberger, K. P., *et al.*: Hodgkin's disease in children. *Cancer*, **31**:560, 1973.

Schwart, D. L., Pierre, R. V., Scheerer, P. P. *et al.*: Lymphosarcoma cell leukemia. *Amer. J. Med.*, **38**:778, 1965.

Singh, A. D. and Scudder, I. B.: Malignancy in childhood. *Indian J. Cancer*, **2**:185, 1965.

Smith, J. L., Barker, C. R., Clein, G. P. *et al.*: Characterization of malignant mediastinal neoplasm (Sternberg Sarcoma) as thymic in origin. *Lancet*, **1**:74, 1973.

Sternberg, C.: Zur renntnis des chloroms (chloromyelosarkom). *Beitr. Pathol. Anat.*, **37**:437, 1905.

Stewart, A. and Kneale, G. W.: Radiation dose effects in obstetric x-rays and childhood cancers. *Lancet*, **1**:1185, 1970.

Stewart, J. K.: Pathology of tumors in children. *J. Clin. Pathol.*, **17**:407, 1964.

Sullivan, M. P.: Leukemic transformation in lymphosarcoma of childhood. *Pediat.*, **29**:589, 1962.

Van Swaay, H.: Aplastic anemia and myeloid leukemia after irradiation of the vertebral column. *Lancet*, **2**:225, 1955.

Wintrobe, M. W.: Clinical Hematology, (Philadelphia: Lea and Febiger, 1961, 940).

CHAPTER 7

Factors which may predispose to lymphoreticular malignancies

The preceeding chapters have emphasised the importance of environmental factors in certain lymphoreticular malignancies and in some instances, a series of hypotheses relating to aetiology have been presented. Thus, Hodgkin's disease might have an infectious component, with an asymptomatic carrier state and a long incubation period. Some prenatal exposure might be essential for the development of Burkitt's lymphoma, a tumour strongly associated with EBV and perhaps malaria in African countries. Childhood Hodgkin's disease and lymphosarcoma might also be induced during the prenatal period, but this is unlikely in reticulum cell sarcoma. There is growing evidence that acute lymphatic leukaemia of childhood might be caused by exposure to a viral agent, possibly varicella, during the prenatal period. Another important concept is that significant epidemiologic, clinical and histologic differences exist between the childhood and adult age groups with certain lymphoreticular malignancies. This is certainly true of Hodgkin's disease and lymphosarcoma and may also apply to acute lymphatic leukaemia. Interestingly all three disorders have bimodal incidence curves, whereas in the majority of instances Burkitt's lymphoma is a disease of childhood and reticulum cell sarcoma occurs in the elderly. This variability makes it unlikely that all of these disorders are due to any one environmental factor; a multiplicity of factors must be involved. Furthermore, in any of these diseases, particularly those with both childhood and adult peaks, it seems quite possible that aetiologic factors exert their influence at different points in time and that the relative importance of certain host factors may vary considerably during these periods.

While at present we must acknowledge our ignorance about both aetiologic and host factors, these considerations can be approached in a limited fashion, by examining possible high risk groups. As will be seen, this frequently results in a fragmentary picture, but the challenge then is to identify the unifying thread that connects all the pieces. This final chapter summarises some of the factors that may be important in predisposing to certain lymphoproliferative malignancies. The listings are by no means complete and most of the factors mentioned require further evaluation. It does, however, represent a starting point.

CHROMOSOMAL ABERRATION AND OTHER GENETIC FACTORS

Table 7.1 lists several different genetic factors which might predispose an individual to the neoplastic disorders indicated. It is well-established that mongols have a 20-fold or greater risk of acute leukaemia (Wald and Borges, 1961). This observation was first made in 1957 by Kirivit and Good and all of the subtypes commonly found in childhood are seen. In contrast to acute childhood leukaemia which peaks around the age of 3 years, the age peak for mongolism associated cases occurs around the first year of life. In addition to frank leukaemia, mongols apparently also have an increased incidence of leukaemoid reactions. It is also interesting that Down's syndrome occurs with increased frequency among sibs of leukaemic children (Miller, 1968). As is true with mongolism, Klinefelter's syndrome, a genetic disorder associated with at least one extra X chromosome, results from meiotic non-disjunction. This disorder has been associated with acute lymphatic (Bousser and Tanzer, 1963), myelogenous (Mamunes *et al.*, 1961), and undifferentiated (Borges *et al.*, 1967) leukaemia, chronic myelogenous leukaemia (Tough *et al.*, 1961) and reticulum cell sarcoma (Augustine and Jaworski, 1958; MacSween, 1965). Further evaluation of this syndrome as a possible predisposing condition is required, since the evidence suggesting an association is based primarily on case reports.

Fanconi's aplastic anaemia and Bloom's syndrome are autosomal recessive disorders characterised by excessive chromosomal breakage. They both appear to be associated with an increased frequency of acute childhood leukaemia, but non-lymphatic types appear to predominate (Bloom *et al.*, 1966; Sawitsky *et al.*, 1966). Additional studies of both syndromes will be required to define the actual risk of leukaemic response. Ataxia-telangiectasia (Louis–Bar syndrome) with an autosomal recessive inheritance pattern and the Wiskott–Aldrich syndrome and Bruton's daammaglobulinaemia, sex-linked recessive disorders, will be considereg further under immune deficiency disorders, but their

Table 7.1 Genetic and racial factors which may predispose to lymphoreticular malignancies

Type	Specific factor	Lymphoreticular malignancy	Association
Chromosome aberration	Down's syndrome	Acute childhood lymphatic leukaemia	Established
	Klinefelter's syndrome	Leukaemia Lymphoma (reticulum cell)	Requires further evaluation
	Congenital chromosomal aneuploidy	Childhood leukaemia	Requires further evaluation
	Chediak–Higashi syndrome	Lymphomas	Probable
	Radiation induced Preconceptional, Prenatal	Acute childhood leukaemia	Probable
	Postnatal	Lymphomas	Requires further evaluation
	Extra band of medium fluorescence chromosome 14q T	Burkitt's lymphoma	Requires further evaluation
Other genetic factors	HL–A System		
	A2, A12	Acute lymphatic leukemia	Requires further evaluation
	4C group-HL–A	Hodgkin's disease	Requires further evaluation
	Identical twins	Increased incidence of acute lymphatic leukaemia if one member has this disease	Requires further evaluation
	Sibs	Aggregation of childhood leukaemia	Probable
Racial			
	Italian, Jewish ancestry	Hodgkin's disease	Requires further evaluation
	Adult white Jewish ancestry, Poles	Leukaemia (chronic lymphatic leukaemia)	Requires further evaluation
	Spanish–American	Higher white cell counts in childhood acute lymphatic leukaemia	Requires further evaluation

primary defect is obviously genetic. The Chediak–Higashi syndrome, an inherited autosomal recessive disorder, is characterised by an alteration in neutrophil morphology and function, the presence of giant lysosomes in these cells, partial albinism, photophobia, nystagmus, and hepatosplenomegaly. While there is no evidence suggesting that this disorder is primarily associated with immune deficiency, it does carry an increased risk of lymphoreticular malignancy (Doll and Kinlen, 1970).

Ionising radiation is a well-established cause of chromosome breakage and it has been suggested that preconceptional or prenatal exposure of parents might increase the risk of acute leukaemia among offspring. A retrospective case–control study of 319 children showed a relative risk of 1·6 and 1·3 respectively for future mothers and fathers following diagnostic radiation (Graham *et al.*, 1966). However, a large prospective study of children by the Atomic Bomb Casualty Commission showed no increase in leukaemia after obviously heavier exposures of parents to preconceptional radiation (Hoshiro *et al.*, 1967). Other studies have indicated that diagnostic radiation during pregnancy increases the risk of childhood leukaemia (Stewart *et al.*, 1956; MacMahon 1962) but Court Brown *et al.*, 1960 failed to confirm this association. In evaluating these studies, it is also important to realise that neither the nature of the chromosomal defect induced nor the type of subsequent neoplastic response attributable to this insult are specific. This seems clear since intra-uterine exposure to radiation appears to be associated with an increased incidence of other childhood malignancies, such as those of the central nervous system. The lack of consistency both in the overall results of the studies mentioned and in the specificity of the neoplastic effect, indicates the need for further study. Particular attention should be given to three related considerations: the possibility that a relationship might exist between maternal preconceptional irradiation and Down's syndrome or other chromosome aberrations (Uchida *et al.*, 1968); the observation that the excess risk of prenatal induced childhood cancer is exhausted by age 8 (MacMahon, 1962); and the evaluation of a possible association between intra-uterine radiation and birth order, since there is a high incidence of leukaemia in first births (MacMahon and Newill, 1962).

Although radiotherapy for conditions such as ankylosing spondylitis is associated with an increased frequency of chronic myelogenous leukaemia (Court Brown and Doll, 1965), there is no apparent increase in the acute or chronic lymphatic varieties. Furthermore, there are no consistent chromosomal abnormalities in either type of lymphatic leukaemia such as the Philadelphia chromosome which is found in chronic myelogenous leukaemia.

The major evidence suggesting an association between radiation and the lymphomas relates to exposure to atomic bombs in Japan, but the results are conflicting when the experience in Hiroshima and Nagasaki are compared (Nishiyama *et al.*, 1973). While it seems possible that such an association might exist, especially for those lymphomas requiring some type of prior immunosuppression this matter will require further evaluation.

Although an extra band of fluorescence has been observed with some frequency on chromosome 14qT in Burkitt's lymphoma (Rowley, 1974), the specific nature of this defect is unknown; that is, it has not been established whether this extra band represents a translocation or a duplication of a chromosomal segment. Although chromosomal abnormalities may be found with some frequency in other lymphomas, there are apparently no characteristic cytogenetic findings for any of these diseases (Spiers and Baikie, 1968).

Still other genetically controlled or related factors appear to have some association with the development of lymphoreticular malignancies (Table 7.1). Several reports have found an increased frequency of the 4C group of the major human histocompatibility antigen system (HL–A system) in Hodgkin's disease (Bodmer 1973). A study of familial Hodgkin's disease (Vianna *et al.*, 1974) has further suggested that host response as measured by the four Rye histologic subtypes might be determined in part by genetic factors. This possibility would appear to be consistent with the observation that HL–A1 and HL–A8 antigens occur more frequently in the mixed cellularity and lymphocyte predominant subtypes (Falk and Osaba, 1971), but not in nodular sclerosis. The fact that certain other studies have failed to demonstrate an association between this lymphoma and the 4C complex however, indicates the need for additional studies. Other reports suggest an association between acute lymphatic leukaemia and HL–A system, the best prognosis being observed in patients with HL–A9. However, all of these observations must be considered as preliminary and require further evaluation. If genetic factors are important in the development of lymphatic leukaemias, family aggregates with these disorders might be observed. An increased frequency of acute lymphatic leukaemia has been observed in twins of similar sex who die before 6 years of age, but not for fraternal twins in the United States (MacMahon and Levy, 1964; Miller, 1968). Unfortunately, these results were not confirmed in Great Britain (Hewitt *et al.*, 1966). It has also been suggested that there is as much as a fourfold excess of leukaemia among the sibs of children with this disorder (Miller, 1968). However, this could be due to environmental or genetic factors or both and it is unclear what subtypes are involved. It has also been suggested that there may be an excess number of familial aggregates of chronic lymphatic leukaemia (Fitzgerald *et al.*, 1966), but this requires substantiation.

Marked differences in the incidence of lymphoreticular malignancies among certain races may be due to genetic factors. In the United States, rates for Hodgkin's disease, other lymphomas and acute childhood leukaemia in whites exceed those for non-whites. Evidence has been presented that the death rate from chronic lymphatic leukaemia in the American Jewish population is approximately twice that in the non-Jewish population (MacMahon and Koller, 1957). Graham and his colleagues (1970) found that Russian Jews had a higher risk than Russians or Jews in general. They also found a higher risk of leukaemia among adults of Polish ancestry but not in children with this or the other ethnic backgrounds mentioned. But observations of this nature might be due to customs specific for these groups or differences in medical care, as Lilienfeld (1959) has suggested. A low overall incidence of leukaemia has been reported among American Negroes over 70 years of age when compared to whites of the same age group (McPhedran *et al.*, 1970). This may be due to socio-economic factors and the availability of medical facilities. In certain oriental populations (Wells and Law, 1960), chronic lymphatic leukaemia is exceedingly rare, and it seems likely that this is due to racial factors. A study conducted by Milham and Hesser, 1967 suggested that Italian surnames appear to be more common among Hodgkin's disease cases, and MacMahon (1966) found a high rate for this disorder among Jews in Brooklyn, New York. Both observations require further substantiation. Knudson (1965) found that the leukaemic response in acute lymphatic leukaemia in childhood differed between Spanish American and non-Spanish American whites; initial white cell counts were rarely less than 10 000 for the former group in contrast to non-Spanish American cases. Since high initial white counts are frequently associated with an unfavourable prognosis, as is HL–A3 histocompatibility antigen (Lawler *et al.*, 1974), it would be interesting to determine whether Spanish American whites (cases and general population) have an increased frequency of this antigen. From what has been said about ethnic differences in various lymphoreticular malignancies, it seems clear that further study of these important findings is indicated. It must be emphasised however, that most of the observations mentioned, while compatible with a genetic interpretation, can also be explained by environmental factors. To realise the full meaning of these differences, we must obviously go beyond initial observations to the reasons behind them.

IMMUNE DEFICIENCY STATES

These represent a heterogeneous group of inborn and acquired defects of the lymphoid system, which may involve the thymic or humoural systems or both (Table 7.2).

Table 7.2 Immune deficiency states which may predispose to lymphoreticular malignancy

Immune deficiency disorder	Specific type	Lymphoreticular malignancy	Association
Congenital disorders	Ataxia telangiectasia	Acute lymphatic leukaemia Hodgkin's disease Lymphosarcoma reticulum cell sarcoma	Requires further evaluation
	Wiskott–Aldrich syndrome	Lymphosarcoma Reticulum cell sarcoma Malignant recticulo-endotheliosis	Established
	Swiss-type agammaglobu-linaemia	Lymphosarcoma Hodgkin's disease	Requires further evaluation
	Bruton-type agammaglobu-linaemia	Acute lymphatic leukaemia	Probable
	Common variable immunodeficiency	'Lymphomas'	Probable
Auto-immune disorders	Sjögren's syndrome	Lymphosarcoma Reticulum cell sarcoma Waldenstrom's macroglobulinaemia	Established
	Rheumatoid arthritis Systemic lupus erythematosis	Malignant lymphomas	Requires further evaluation
Induced immune disorders	Organ transplantation with immune suppression	Reticulum cell sarcoma	Established

Congenital immunologic disorders

An emerging concept in recent years is that the lymphoreticular malignancies are associated with immunodeficiency states in man and lower animals. If the immune system in certain animals is suppressed, either by surgical means such as thymectomy or by immunosuppressive drugs, it becomes considerably easier to induce tumours. It comes as no surprise that in man, patients with primary deficiencies of their immune systems have a high incidence of lymphomas and lymphatic leukaemia (Good, 1972).

Ataxia-telangiectasia is characterised by progressive cerebellar ataxia, telangiectasia of the skin and conjunctiva and frequent sino-pulmonary infection. Genetically it is an autosomal recessive disorder and chromosome fragility can be demonstrated on cell culture. Immunologic deficiency is manifested by low serum IgA levels, hypoplastic thymic and lymphoid tissues and impaired delayed hypersensitivity and lymphocyte transformation. Approximately 10 per cent of patients with this disorder develop a malignant disease (Waldmann *et al.*, 1972), and in most instances the tumours are lymphomas or lymphatic leukaemia. For example, reticulum cell sarcoma in a 27-month-old child with this syndrome (Feigen *et al.*, 1970), Hodgkin's disease in a 4-year-old child (Harris and Seeler, 1973) and acute leukaemia in three children, among which two were sibs with the lymphatic subtype, (Hecht *et al.*, 1966) have been described. A third sib in this family also had ataxia-telangiectasia and laboratory studies on this child demonstrated a high frequency of chromosomal breaks and an impaired lymphocyte response to phytohaemagglutinin. It will be important to determine whether the deficient immunoglobulin production and qualitative lymphocyte defect can be found in individuals without the characteristic clinical features of this syndrome.

The Wiskott–Aldrich syndrome is a sex-linked recessive immune disorder characterised by hypoplastic thymic and lymphoid tissue, a decrease in IgM immunoglobulin levels and an impaired delayed-hypersensitivity response. Cooper *et al.* (1968) has suggested that the basic defect of this disorder is an inability to process polysaccharide antigens with a resulting chronic antigenic stimulation. Clinically the syndrome is characterised by the triad of thrombocytopenia, eczema and frequent infection. Several instances have been described where this disorder has been associated with lymphomas (Doll and Kinlen, 1970).

In the Swiss type of agammaglobulinaemia there is an increased tendency for a variety of infections and lymphomas such as Hodgkin's disease and lymphosarcoma. As is true for ataxia-telangiectasia, these lymphomas can develop at a very early age. Bruton's X-linked agamma-globulinaemia is characterised by a defect in humoural immunity and an increased frequency of lymphatic leukaemia (Good *et al.*, 1970). Page *et al.* (1963) studied twenty-four children with congenital agamma-globulinaemia and found that one developed a lymphoma and another, acute lymphatic leukaemia. Further study of this disorder and its possible association with lymphomas is required. The common variable disorder is often genetically determined, and is characterised by defects in B- and T-lymphocyte function. This condition is frequently associated with auto-immune manifestations, intestinal nodular lymphoid hyper-plasia and probably an increased frequency of lymphomas (Medical Research Council Working Party, 1969). However, if some association does exist, it does not appear to be specific since other malignant dis-orders have been found among cases with this immunodeficiency. In contrast to the congenital immunologic deficiency states described above, no cases of lymphoma have been described in DiGeorge syndrome, which is characterised by a congenital failure in thymus development. However, this might be due to the fact that such patients die at an early age.

Auto-immune disorders

Although lymphomas have been reported among patients with various auto-immune disorders including lupus erythematosis, the possibility that such an association exists has not been evaluated sufficiently. The rarity of these collagen vascular disorders and the frequent lack of specific criteria in establishing their diagnosis, undoubtedly make such studies difficult to conduct. As mentioned previously (Chapter 4), results may be difficult to interpret since these auto-immune disorders may mimic the lymphomas clinically. Furthermore, disorders such as rheumatoid arthritis, which can produce lymphofollicular hyperplasia, must be distinguished from lymphomas of the giant follicular type (Rappaport, 1966). Another possibility that must be considered is that the various rheumatoid disorders might be the result of an underlying lymphoma in certain instances. Thus, Nosanchuk and Schnitzer (1969) reviewed a number of cases of Hodgkin's disease, lymphosarcoma and histiocytic sarcoma in patients with rheumatoid arthritis and in all instances these malignancies were present at the time of initial biopsy. Despite these limitations, the numerous case reports suggesting an association, and the fact that there are several experimental examples where auto-immunity is associated with lymphoid neoplasia (e.g. aleutian disease) make clear the need for further study of a possible association between the auto-immune disorders and lymphoreticular malignancies. In contrast to the other auto-immune disorders, available evidence suggests that Sjögren's syndrome does predispose to lymphomas (Cummings *et al.*, 1971). This syndrome occurs primarily in middle-aged females and is associated with a spectrum of lymphoid involvement, ranging from lymphocyte infiltration of the salivary glands and other organs to frank lymphoreticular malignancy. This observation and the facts that half the patients with Sjögren's syndrome have rheumatoid arthritis while others may have lupus erythematosis, polyarteritis and polymyositis, raise the possibility that all of these disorders may have some common defect which predisposes to lymphoma. It will also be important to determine if any of the collagen vascular diseases alone are associated with an elevated frequency of lymphoreticular malignancy or is the combination of one of these disorders and immunosuppressive therapy required. In view of the established association between reticulum cell sarcoma and immunosuppression in organ transplant cases, this latter possibility must be considered. The association between organ transplantation and malignant lymphomas has been discussed previously (Chapter 4) and reviewed by Penn and Starzl (1972). These investigators studied the malignant tumours arising in seventy-five patients who survived organ transplants for long periods and found twenty cases of reticulum cell sarcoma, four unclassified lymphomas, three cases with Kaposi's sarcoma and one with lymphosarcoma. Of more than passing interest is the fact that Kaposi's sarcoma can itself be considered as a predisposing factor to lymphoreticular tumours, especially Hodgkin's disease (Moertel, 1966; Templeton, 1972).

BIRTH ASSOCIATED FACTORS

The possibility that newborn humans might be as susceptible to leukaemogenic influences as laboratory animals, has led the epidemiologist to consider whether various birth related factors might be important in this disorder. It is likely that a higher than expected proportion of first births occur among leukaemic children and that they have older mothers (Table 7.3). MacMahon and Newill (1962) demonstrated that the maternal-age and birth-order effects were mutually indepen-

Table 7.3 Birth associated factors which may predispose to certain lymphoreticular malignancies

Factor	Lymphoreticular malignancy	Status
Older mothers	Acute childhood (lymphatic?) leukaemia	Established
Below average birth order	Acute childhood (lymphatic?) leukaemia	Established
High birth weight	Acute childhood (lymphatic?) leukaemia	Established
Birth month	Acute childhood lymphatic leukaemia	Requires further evaluation
	Childhood Hodgkin's disease	Probable

dent. They suggested further that the birth-order effect, but not maternal-age, varied with age at death from leukaemia. Stark and Mantel (1969) presented data which suggested that the birth-order effect was strongest for leukaemia deaths in the third through tenth years of life, that the maternal-age effect was strongest in the fourth through eighth years of life and little association existed between these factors and the risk of acute myelocytic leukaemia in childhood. This latter observation does not mean *de facto* that these birth characteristics are associated with acute lymphatic leukaemias alone, for this cell type has many characteristics in common with the undifferentiated variety, despite the fact that recent evidence suggests that the two varieties may differ aetiologically. Thus, the first question, in the way of defining the association between birth order, maternal-age and childhood leukaemia, is whether these factors related to one or both of these subtypes. If we assume for the moment that these factors predispose to acute lymphatic leukaemia, on the grounds that this cell type accounts for the majority of cases under 10 years of age, how might they be explained? One explanation might be that maternal gametes or the *in utero* environment differs in young and older females. This, however, would not explain the birth-order effect which is independent of maternal age. Another hypothesis would be to evoke some environmental factor, possibly a viral disease. Of necessity this viral disease must have at least three characteristics: it must be capable of being triggered off by pregnancy regardless of maternal age; it must be more common in the later years of child-bearing; and it must confer prolonged immunity after the first exposure. Thus, the offspring of the comparatively older female experiencing her first pregnancy would have a high risk as would the first born of any female or a child whose mother was old at pregnancy. Without lasting immunity, one might expect most pregnancies to have a similar risk. Perhaps the best example of a viral disease with the three characteristics mentioned is herpes zoster. This agent is identical serologically to varicella, which has already been implicated as a possible cause of acute lymphatic leukaemia in childhood. Clinically, zoster infection occurs most frequently in overworked persons and it has been specifically associated with the pregnant state. The incidence of this disorder increases with age and second attacks are exceedingly rare. There are undoubtedly other possible explanations for the two birth characteristics mentioned above, but in all likelihood their association with childhood leukaemia will ultimately be explained by some environmental influence.

Considering other possible birth associated factors, high birth weight (Table 7.3) has been found to be associated with an increased risk of childhood leukaemia, especially in females (MacMahon and Newill, 1962). This is not surprising since birth weight is known to vary with race, birth order, maternal age and social class, all factors thought to affect the risk of leukaemia. One of the most informative birth associated features is seasonality by month of birth, an observation which is compatible with the activity of an environmental factor around the time of birth and/or during the prenatal period. As mentioned in Chapter 5, there have been several attempts to demonstrate seasonality in childhood leukaemia but few studies have examined individual subtypes and urban-rural factors. Preliminary evidence does suggest that various age groups of acute lymphatic leukaemia in urban counties might have different seasonality by month of birth, but this will require further study. If confirmed, it will provide strong additional evidence that environmental factors are important in this disorder. A similar approach should be taken with childhood lymphosarcoma since it is well-established that leukaemic transformation occurs most frequently with this particular lymphoma. Are there different types of acute lymphatic leukaemia, some of which are closely related to childhood lymphosarcoma? It has already been mentioned that undifferentiated and T(thymic) varieties of childhood lymphatic leukaemia have been identified. Seasonality by month of birth has been observed for childhood Hodgkin's disease. Fraumeni and Li (1969) in a study of 359 death certificates of United States children who died of Hodgkin's disease, observed a birth month seasonality (i.e. among boys dying of this disorder, a higher than expected number were born in July and

August). Urban-rural factors were not considered in this important study, but in view of the reported high incidence of Hodgkin's disease in male children from rural regions, it seems possible that the strength of the seasonality observed might lie in this type of area. Studies of seasonality by month of birth should be assigned a very high priority. They must however, be sufficiently large to consider important factors such as age, sex, specific histologic types of the lymphoreticular disorders and urban–rural differences.

OCCUPATIONAL–SOCIAL FACTORS

If environmental factors are as important in most of lymphoreticular malignancies, occupational studies must be considered to be important potential sources of information. Milham and Hesser (1967) found an association between occupations involving exposure to wood and Hodgkin's disease (Table 7.4). Although two other reports (Vianna *et al.*, 1971; Acheson 1967) failed to confirm this association, one of these

Table 7.4 Occupational and social factors which may predispose to lymphoreticular malignancies

Specific factor	Lymphoreticular malignancy	Association
Occupational		
Woodworkers	Hodgkin's disease	Requires further evaluation
Young male farmers	Hodgkin's disease	Requires further evaluation
Chemists (male)	lymphomas	Requires further evaluation
Anaesthesiologists	Non-Hodgkin's lymphomas	Requires further evaluation
Physicians (male)	Hodgkin's disease	Requires further evaluation
Teachers (male)	Hodgkin's disease	Requires further evaluation
Social		
High social class	Hodgkin's disease	Probable (age-dependent)
	Other lymphomas	Requires further evaluation
	Acute childhood leukaemia	Probable

studies dealt with patients 40 years or less only and, therefore, no comment could be made about the elderly. Furthermore, Spiers (1969) found marked interstate variations in male mortality due to Hodgkin's disease east of the Rocky Mountains of the United States. These variations in rate appeared to correlate well with the proportion of people working with wood and to the percentage of pine forests in each state. However, this association was not observed in western states. Additional studies of incidence of Hodgkin's disease in woodworkers, especially in older age groups, are needed. If this relationship is verified, it would be most helpful to determine whether any specific group, among those who work in the wood industry, have an excessively high risk.

Fasal and his colleagues (1968) found that the mortality and incidence rates for Hodgkin's disease were higher at younger ages among Californian male farm residents. Similar observations were made for Norwegian male rural residents and it is therefore difficult to determine whether these high rates are due to occupational or urban–rural differences. Other studies have suggested that a high frequency of lymphomas might occur among chemists (Li *et al.*, 1969), anaethesiologists (Bruce *et al.*, 1968), physicians (Vianna *et al.*, 1974), and teachers (Milham, 1974). Each of these associations are based on singular reports and therefore require further evaluation (Table 7.4). Histologic reassessment should be an important component of future studies since it may well be that certain exposures increase the risk of developing only a specific type of lymphoreticular malignancy.

In general, mortality ratios in upper social classes appear to be high for most of the lymphoreticular malignancies in western countries (Table 7.4). In England and Wales from 1949–53 the standard mortality ratios for lymphomas and leukaemia among males and married females were highest for those belonging to the highest social class (class 1) (MacMahon, 1966). During this same period, the highest average annual death rates from Hodgkin's disease were also observed for this group and this association between mortality and social class was seen in each age group in each sex. From 1959–63, however, similar results were not observed (Registrar-General's Decennial Supplement), and in Manchester from 1962–65 (Alderson and Nayak, 1972) no significant social class variation was found for men diagnosed with Hodgkin's disease. In New York State the mortality rate for Hodgkin's disease in high socio-economic counties does appear to be slightly (but not significantly) higher than that for the state as a whole (Vianna *et al.*, 1974). In the

United States, the incidence of Hodgkin's disease was reported to be lowest among World War II white male recruits from a low social class, based on their pre-service occupation (Cohen *et al.*, 1964). However, that there is a specific association between high social class and the incidence of various lymphoreticular malignancies is not fully established at present, for as MacMahon (1966) has pointed out, socio-economic status is closely related to other variables such as duration of education, intelligence and occupational class. In the study conducted by Cohen *et al.* (1964), World War II soldiers with Hodgkin's disease tended to be of above average intelligence and to come from occupations that required a high degree of intelligence. All of these factors should be considered in future epidemiologic studies.

PRIOR INFECTION

This is a very difficult category to evaluate properly, since even where a strong association between some prior infection and a particular lymphoreticular malignancy is demonstrated, one must question whether the infection is merely an early manifestation of the underlying disease. For example, Kneale's study (1971) stresses the sensitivity of pre-leukaemics to pneumonia, a common cause of death in children. Table 7.5 lists the infectious diseases and lymphoreticular malignancies with which they might be related. The evidence suggesting an association between varicella, influenza, EBV and malaria and various neoplastic disorders is based on formal epidemiologic studies, which have been described in previous chapters. A series of case reports form the basis for the other disorders listed. Thus, one report (Andrade and Abreu, 1971) described eight cases of follicular lymphoma of the spleen in patients with hepatosplenic schistosomiasis mansoni (Andrade and Abreu, 1971). Another study presented information on six patients with leprosy who developed malignant lymphomas, particularly Hodgkin's disease and lymphoblastic lymphoma (Rodriquez *et al.*, 1968). In all instances, the lymphomas appeared many years after the onset of leprosy (range 10–22 years). One can speculate that if this latter association is real, it might be due to some aberration in the host's immune status. In keeping with this possibility, is the observation of a higher prevalence of auto-antibodies among leprosy patients than controls (Petchclai *et al.*, 1973). Among eighty-six cases of acute toxoplasmic lymphadenitis, Morgenfeld (1974) observed one case of lymphocytic

Table 7.5 Infectious agents which might predispose to lymphoreticular malignancies

Infectious disease (or agent)	Lymphoreticular malignancy	Association
(Congenital) Varicella	Acute (lymphatic) leukaemia in childhood	Requires further evaluation
(Congenital) Influenza	Acute childhood leukaemia Hodgkin's disease	Requires further evaluation
Epstein–Barr virus	Burkitt's lymphoma (Africa) Hodgkin's disease	Requires further evaluation
Malaria	Burkitt's lymphoma (Africa)	Requires further evaluation
Schistosomiasis mansoni	Follicular lymphoma	Requires further evaluation
Leprosy	Lymphoblastic lymphoma Hodgkin's disease	Requires further evaluation
Toxoplasma gondii	Lymphocytic lymphoma Chronic lymphatic leukaemia	Requires further evaluation
Feline leukaemia virus	Acute leukaemia Lymphoma	Requires further evaluation

lymphoma and a case of chronic lymphatic leukaemia. All of these observations are preliminary in nature, but the possibility that the infectious diseases mentioned might act as predisposing factors to certain lymphatic malignancies must be evaluated further.

A few comments about EBV infectious mononucleosis are warranted. A possible association between this disorder and some lymphatic neoplasms has been a matter of great speculation, and some have suggested that mononucleosis might be a self-limited form of neoplasia. In the past particular attention has been given to the possible relationship of infectious mononucleosis and acute lymphatic leukaemia. The results of clinical, epidemiologic and serologic studies all suggest that a causal relationship does not exist between the two disorders. While infectious mononucleosis can precede leukaemia, it can also occur at various stages during haematologic remission (*Lancet* editorial, 1971; Freedman *et al.*, 1970). Fraumeni (1971) conducted a case–control study which suggested that a history of mononucleosis was as frequent among leukaemic children as among controls. Furthermore, a prospective study of EBV in children with acute lymphatic leukaemia indicated that five of twelve untreated patients had no serologic evidence of infection at the onset or during the course of their malignancy (Miller *et al.*, 1972). Interestingly, mononucleosis may occasionally ameliorate the clinical course of leukaemia (Stevens *et al.*, 1971).

Animal contact

The viral aetiology of leukaemia in chickens, mice and cats is well-established, and there is strong evidence implicating a C-type virus-like agent in bovine leukaemia. These facts raise the question whether these and other animals represent a zoonotic hazard to man? The occurrence of similar lymphoreticular malignancies in man and domestic or farm animals with whom he has had contact (Heath, 1970) adds some support to this possibility, but one must determine whether these events are related merely by chance. Feline and canine leukaemia and lymphoma are not rare disorders; in fact Dorn *et al.* (1967) have suggested that combined rates for these animals are higher than those for man and the feline rate is about $2\frac{1}{2}$ times greater. Male cats have a higher risk of malignant lymphoma than female cats (Dorn *et al.*, 1968), as is true for humans. It should also be noted that the oncogenic activity of feline leukaemia virus can be transmitted to other species including dogs (Rickard *et al.*, 1973), and that this agent can grow in cultured human cells (Sarma *et al.*, 1970). Overall rates for bovine leukaemia (or lymphosarcoma) are not known, but this is the most common tumour of dairy cattle and it tends to occur in familial and herd aggregations (Marshak *et al.*, 1962). This disorder also has many pathologic features in common with lymphosarcoma in man.

The epidemiology of cat leukaemia and its possible relationship to man has been the subject of many studies. In addition to what has already been mentioned, we know that the feline leukaemia virus can be found in the saliva and urine of diseased cats (Gardner *et al.*, 1971), that many healthy cats give serologic evidence of exposure to this virus and clusters of cat leukaemia have been described in households (Hardy *et al.*, 1973). While these observations indicate the ease with which humans might be exposed to cat leukaemia virus, the major question remains: are humans at increased risk of leukaemia or lymphoma because of such exposure? The majority of epidemiologic evidence at present suggests that this is not the case. Two studies of veterinarians (Fasal *et al.*, 1966; Botts *et al.*, 1966) as a possible risk group yielded negative results with respect to the lymphoreticular malignancies. Furthermore, a serologic survey suggests that cat virus antibody is rarely found in veterinarians (Schneider and Riggs, 1973). Schneider *et al.*, (1968) identified over 400 households with cases of animal neoplasia and found no significant cancer when these households were compared with matched control households. Schneider (1970; 1972) conducted two case–control studies, one dealing with all feline neoplasia and the other specifically with feline lymphoma and found no significant difference between case and control households. Another study of leukaemic and lymphomatous children and controls (Van Hoosier *et al.*, 1968) found no significant difference in the frequency of contact with dogs for this group when compared to controls. But not all studies have been negative for Bross *et al.* (1970, 1972) reported a positive correlation between cases of acute leukaemia and exposure to sick pets. There are two aspects of these studies which will be important to consider in future investigations: relative risks were found to be highly significant when exposure to 'sick' cats occurred; and in the childhood study, when sickness or death of cats during the period from the birth of the child was considered the relative risk increased from 1·35 to 2·24. Despite the fact that most of the studies of possible feline–human lymphoreticular malignancy have been negative, the possibility that some association exists must be considered further. If some form of transmission does occur, it may be intermittent and the time of hypothetical exposure may be of great importance. It will undoubtedly require the combined efforts of the veterinarians, epidemiologist, immunologist and virologist to finally resolve this matter.

OTHER FACTORS

The possible association between hydantoin or amphetamine ingestion and various malignant lymphomas has already been mentioned (Chapter 4). The evidence that prior tonsillectomy might be a predisposing factor in Hodgkin's disease was presented in Chapter 2. All of these considerations require further evaluation.

Of the many possible predisposing factors mentioned, some will undoubtedly be excluded, only to be replaced by others. It will be important therefore, to constantly evaluate each new lead for a thread of consistency both with other potential influencing factors and the overall hypotheses under consideration. For the present, a few generalisations might be made cautiously. Immune deficiency states, be they congenital or acquired, genetic or environmental, seem to be associated with an increased risk of lymphatic leukaemia or lymphoma. The two disorders for which birth associated factors have been identified (Table 7.3), have bimodal incidence curves. It will be interesting to determine whether these or other factors of this type are associated with the childhood peak of lymphosarcoma. The possibility that exposure to radiation might enhance ones risk of developing a lymphoreticular malignancy, particularly histiocytic lymphoma, is consistent with the concept that factors capable of altering the immune response can predispose to this group of disorders. Admittedly there is no specific neoplastic response associated with this exposure, but this is also absent in transplant patients. Chemists and anaesthesiologists, by the very nature of their occupations, are chronically exposed to potentially toxic substances, some of which might be capable of immunosuppression. If these associations (Table 7.4) are confirmed, specific chemicals should be evaluated for this property. In the case of farmers, physicians and teachers, the important exposure may be in the form of animal or human contact. All of these potential associations must be underlined by the factor of time for it is clear that ageing alters immunity and the same stimulus can result in totally different responses in the young and old.

References

Acheson, E. D.; Hodgkin's disease in woodworkers. *Lancet*, **2**:988, 1967.

Alderson, M. R. and Nayak, R.: Epidemiology of Hodgkin's disease. *J. Chronic. Dis.*, **25**:253, 1972.

Andrade, Z. A. and Abreu, W. N.: Follicular lymphoma of the spleen in patients with hepatosplenic schistosomiasis mansoni. *Amer. J. Trop. Med. Hyg.*, **20**:237, 1971.

Augustine, J. R. and Jaworski, Z. F.; Unusual testicular histology in true Klinefelter's syndrome. *Arch. Pathol.*, **66**:159, 1958.

Bloom, G. E., Warner, S., Gerald, P. S. *et al.*: Chromosome abnormalities in constitutional aplastic anemia. *New Eng. J. Med.*, **274**:8, 1966.

Bodmer, W. F.: Genetic factors in Hodgkin's disease: association with a disease-susceptibility locus (DSA) in the HL–A region. In: *International Symposium on Hodgkin's Disease*, 36 Washington, D.C.: (U.S. Government Printing Office, 1972, 127) (National Cancer Institute Monograph).

Borges, W. H., Nichlas, J. W. and Hamm, C. W.: Prezygotic determinants in acute leukemia. *J. Pediat.*, **70**:180, 1967.

Botts, R. P., Edlavitch, S. and Payne, G.: Mortality in Missouri veterinarians. *J.A.V.M.A.*, **149**:499, 1966.

Bousser, J. and Tanzer, J.: Syndrome det Klinefelter et leucemié aigue, a propos d'um cas. *Nouv. Rev. Franc. Hematol.*, **3**:194, 1963.

Bross, I. D., Bertell, R. and Gibson, R.: Pets and adult leukemia. *Amer. J. Pub. Health*, **62**:1520, 1972.

Bross, I. D. and Gibson, R., Cats and childhood leukemia. *J. Med. (Basel)*, **1**:180, 1970.

Bruce, D. L., Eide, K. A., Linde, H. W. *et al.*: Causes of death among anesthesiologists: a 20 year survey. *Anesthesiology*, **29**:565, 1968.

Cohen, B. M., Smetana, H. F. and Miller, R. W.: Hodgkin's disease: long survival in a study of 388 World War II army cases. *Cancer*, **17**:856, 1964.

Cooper, M. D., Chae, H. P., Lowman, J. T. *et al.*: Wiskott–Aldrich syndrome:

an immunologic deficiency disease involving the afferent limb of immunity. *Amer. J. Med.*, **44**:499, 1968.

Court Brown, W. M. and Doll, R.: Mortality from cancer and other causes after radiotherapy for ankylosing spondylitis. *Brit. Med. J.*, **2**:1327, 1965.

Court Brown, W. M., Doll, R. and Hill, A. B.: The incidence of leukemia following exposure to diagnostic radiation *in utero. Brit. Med. J.*, **2**:1539, 1960.

Cummings, N. A., Schall, G. L. and Asofsky, R.: Sjögrens syndrome–newer aspects of research, diagnosis and therapy. *Ann. Int. Med.*, **75**:937, 1971.

Doll, R. and Kinlen, L.: Immunosurveillance and cancer: epidemiological evidence. *Brit. Med. J.*, **4**:420, 1970.

Dorn, C. R., Taylor, D. O. N. and Gibbard, H. H.: Epizoetiologic characteristics of canine and feline leukemia and lymphoma. *Amer. J. Vet. Res.*, **28**:993, 1967.

Dorn, C. R., Taylor, D. O. N., Schneider, R. *et al.*: Survey of animal neoplasms in Alameda and Contra Costa Counties, California. 11. *J. Nat. Cancer Inst.*, **40**:307, 1968.

Essex, M., Cotter, S. O. M. and Carpenter, J. L.: Feline virus induced tumors and the immune response: recent developments. *Amer. J. Vet Res.*, **34**:809, 1973.

Falk, J. and Osoba, D.: HL–A anitgens and survival in Hodgkin's disease. *Lancet*, **2**:1118, 1971.

Fasal, E., Jackson, E. W. and Klauber, M. R.: Mortality in California veterinarians. *J. Chron. Dis.*, **19**:293, 1968.

Feigen, R. D., Vietti, T. J., Wyatt, R. G. *et al.*: Ataxia-telangiectasia with granulocytopenia. *J. Pediat.*, **77**:431, 1970.

Fitzgerald, P. H., Crossen, P. E., Adams, A. C. *et al.*: Chromosome studies in familial leukemia. *J. Med. Genet.*, **3**:96, 1966.

Fraumeni, J. F.: Infectious mononucleosis and acute leukemia. *J.A.M.A.*, **215**:1159, 1971.

Fraumeni, J. F. and Li, F. P.: Hodgkin's disease in childhood: an epidemiological study. *J. Nat. Cancer Inst.*, **42**:681, 1969.

Freedman, M. H., Gilchrist, G. S. and Hammond, G. D.: Concurrent infectious mononucleosis and acute leukemia. *J.A.M.A.*, **217**:1677, 1970.

Gardner, M. B., Rongery, R. W., Johnson, E. Y. *et al.*: C-type tumor virus particles in salivary tissue of domestic house cats. *J. Nat. Cancer Inst.*, **47**:561, 1971.

Good, R. A.: Relations between immunity and malignancy. *Proc. Nat. Acad. Sci. (USA)*, **69**:1026, 1972.

Good, R. A., Finstad, J. and Gatti, R. A.: Bulwarks of the bodily defense. In: *Infectious Agents and Host Reactions*, 76 (S. Mudd, editor) (Philadelphia: W. B. Saunders Co, 1970).

Graham, S., Gibson, R., Lilienfeld, A. *et al.*: Religion and ethnicity in leukemia. *Amer. J. Pub. Health*, **66**:266, 1970.

Graham, S., Levin, M. L., Lilienfeld, A. M. *et al.*: Preconceptional intrauterine and postnatal irradiation as related to leukemia. *Nat. Cancer Inst. Monograph*, **19**:347, 1966.

Hardy, W. D., Old, L. J., Hess, P. W. *et al.*: Horizontal transmission of feline leukemia virus. *Nature (London)*, **244**:266, 1973.

Harris, V. J. and Seeler, R. A.: Ataxia-telangiectasia and Hodgkin's disease. *Cancer*, **32**:1415, 1973.

Heath, C. W., Jr: Human leukemia: genetic and environmental clusters. In: *Comparative Leukemia Research*, 649 (R. M. Dutcher, editor) (1970).

Hecht, F., Koler, R. D., Rigas, D. A. *et al.*: Leukemia and lymphocytes in ataxia-telangiectasia. *Lancet*, **2**:1193, 1966.

Hewitt, D., Lashof, J. C. and Stewart, A. M.: Childhood cancer in twins. *Cancer*, **19**:157, 1966.

Hoshiro, T., Kato, H., Finch, S. C. *et al.*: Leukemia in offspring of atomic bomb survivors. *Blood*, **30**:719, 1967.

Kirivit, W. and Good, R. A.: Simulteneous occurrence of mongolism and leukemia: a report of a nationwide survey. *Amer. J. Dis. Child*, **94**:289, 1957.

Kneale, G. W.: Excess sensitivity of pre-leukaemics to pneumonia: a model situation for studying the interaction of infectious disease with cancer. *Brit. J. Prev. Soc. Med.*, **25**:152, 1971.

Knudson, A. G.: Ethnic differences in childhood leukemia as revealed by a study of antecedent variables. *Cancer*, **18**:815, 1965.

Lancet, Editorial: Infectious mononucleosis and acute leukemia. **1**, 688, 1971.

Lawler, S. D., Klouda, P. T., Smith, P. G. *et al.*: Survival and the HL–A system in acute lymphoblastic leukemia. *Brit. Med. J.*, **1**:547, 1974.

Li, F., Fraumeni, J. F., Mantel, N. *et al.*: Cancer mortality among chemists. *J. Nat. Cancer Inst.*, **43**:1159, 1969.

Lilienfeld, A. M.: Diagnostic and theraputic x-radiation in an urban population. **74**:29, 1959.

MacMahon, B.: Prenatal x-ray exposure and childhood cancer. *J. Nat. Cancer Inst.*, **28**:1173, 1962.

MacMahon, B. and Newill, V. A.: Birth characteristics of children dying of malignant neoplasms. *J. Nat. Cancer Inst.*, **28**:231, 1962.

MacMahon, B.: Epidemiology of Hodgkin's disease. *Cancer Res.*, **26**:1189, 1966.

MacMahon, B. and Koller, E. K.: Ethnic differences in the incidence of leukemia. *Blood*, **12**:1, 1957.

MacMahon, B., Levy, M. A.: Prenatal origin of childhood leukemia: Evidence from twins. *New Eng. J. Med.*, **270**:1082, 1964.

MacSween, R. N. M.: Reticulum cell sarcoma and rheumatoid arthritis in a patient with XY/XXY/XXXY Klinefelter's syndrome and normal intelligence. *Lancet*, **1**:460, 1965.

Mamunes, P., Lapidus, P. H., Abbott, J. A. *et al.*: Acute leukemia and Klinefelter's syndrome. *Lancet*, **2**:26, 1961.

Marshak, R. R., Coriell, L. L., Lawrence, W. C. *et al.*: Studies on bovine lymphosarcoma. I. Clinical aspects, pathological alterations, and herd studies. *Cancer Res.*, **22**:202, 1962.

McPhedran, P., Heath, C. and Garcia, J. S.: Racial variation in leukemia incidence among the elderly. *J. Nat. Cancer Inst.*, **45**:25, 1970.

Medical Research Council Working Party: Hypogammaglobulinemia in the United Kingdom. *Lancet*, **1**:163, 1969.

Milham, S.: Hodgkin's disease as an occupational disease of schoolteachers. *New Eng. J. Med.*, **290**:1329, 1974.

Milham, S. and Hesser, J.: Hodgkin's disease in woodworkers. *Lancet*, **2**:136, 1967.

Miller, G., Shope, T., Heston, L. *et al.*: Prospective study of Epstein–Barr virus infections in acute lymphoblastic leukemia of childhood. *J. Pediat.*, **80**:932, 1972.

Miller, R. W.: Deaths from childhood cancer in sibs. *New Eng. J. Med.*, **279**:122, 1968.

Moertel, C. G.: Multiple primary malignant neoplasms. Their incidence and significance. In: *Recent Results in Cancer Research*, 44 (P.Rentchnick, editor) (Berlin, Heidelberg, New York: Springer-Verlag, 1966) .

Morgenfeld, M. C.: Toxoplasmosis. *Medicina*, **34**:48, 1974.

Nishiyama, H., Anderson, R. E., Ishimaru, T. *et al*.: The incidence of malignant lymphoma and multiple myeloma in Hiroshima and Nagasaki atomic bomb survivors. *Cancer*, **32**:1301, 1973.

Nosanchuk, J. S. and Schnitzer, B.: Follicular hyperplasia in lymph nodes from patients with rheumatoid arthritis. *Cancer*, **24**:343, 1969.

Page, A. R., Hansen, A. E. and Good, R. A.: Occurrence of leukemia and lymphoma in patients with agammaglobulinemia. *Blood*, **21**:197, 1963.

Penn, I. and Starzl, T. E.: Malignant tumors arising *de novo* in immunosuppressed organ transplant recipients. *Transplantation*, **14**:407, 1972.

Petchclai, B., Chuthanondh, R., Rungruong, S. *et al*.: Autoantibodies in leprosy among Thai patients. *Lancet*, **1**:1481, 1973.

Rappaport, H.: Tumors of the hematopoietic system. In: *Atlas of Tumor Pathology*, Sect. III, Fasc. (Washington, D.C.: Armed Forces Institute of Pathology, 1966).

Rickard, C. G., Post, J. E., Noranha, F. *et al*.: Feline tumor viruses. In: *Biohazards in Biologic Research: Proceedings of a Conference on Biohazards in Cancer Research*, 166 (A. Hellman, M. N. Oxman and R. Pollack, editors). (New York, Cold Spring Harbor, 1973).

Rodriquez, E., deBonaparte, Y. P., Morgenfeld, M. C. *et al*.: Malignant lymphomas in leprosy patients—a clinical and histopathologic study. *Int. J. Leprosy*, **36**:203, 1968.

Rowley, J. D.: Do human tumors show a chromosome pattern specific for each etiologic agent? *J. Nat. Cancer Inst.*, **52**:315, 1974.

Sarma, P. S., Huebner, R. J., Basker, J. F. *et al*.: Feline leukemia and sarcoma virus: susceptibility of human cells to infection. *Science*, **168**:1098, 1970.

Sawitsky, A., Bloom, D. and German, J.: Chromosomal breakage and acute leukemia in congenital telangiectatic erythema and stunted growth. *Ann. Int. Med.*, **65**:487, 1966.

Schneider, R.: The natural history of malignant lymphoma and sarcoma in cats and their associations with cancer in man and dog. *J.A.V.M.A.*, `157`: 1753, 1970.

Schneider, R.: Human cancer in households containing cats with malignant lymphoma. *Int. J. Cancer*, **10**:338, 1972.

Schneider, R., Dorn, C. R. and Klauber, M. R.: Cancer in households: a human–canine retrospective study. *J. Nat. Cancer Inst.*, **41**:1285, 1968.

Schneider, R. and Riggs, J. L.: A serologic survey for antibody to feline leukemia virus. *J.A.V.M.A.*, **162**:217, 1973.

Spiers, P. S.: Hodgkin's disease in workers in the wood industry. *Pub. Health Rep.*, **84**:385, 1969.

Spiers, A. and Baikie, A.: Cytogenetic studies in malignant lymphomas and related neoplasms: results in 27 cases. *Cancer*, **22**:193, 1968.

Stark, C. R. and Mantel, N.: Maternal-age and birth-order effects in childhood leukemia: age of child and type of leukemia. *J. Nat. Cancer Inst.*, **42**:857, 1969.

Stevens, D. A., Levine, P. H., Lee, S. K. *et al*.: Concurrent infectious mononucleosis and acute leukemia. *Amer. J. Med.*, **50**:208, 1971.

Stewart, A., Webb, J., Giles, D. *et al*.: Malignant disease in childhood and diagnostic irradiation *in utero*: preliminary communication. *Lancet*, **2**:447, 1956.

Templeton, A. C.: Studies in Kaposi's sarcoma: postmortem findings and disease patterns in women. *Cancer*, **30**:854, 1972.

The Registrar-General's Decennial Supplement, England and Wales, 1961. Occupational mortality tables, 418 (London, H.M.S.O., 1971).

Tough, I. M., Court Brown, W. M., Baikie, A. G. *et al.*: Cytogenic studies in chronic myeloid leukemia and acute leukemia associated with mongolism. *Lancet*, **1**:411, 1961.

Uchida, I. A., Holunga, R and Lawler, C.: Maternal radiation and chromosomal aberrations. *Lancet*, **2**:1045, 1968.

Van Hoosier, G. L., Stenback, W. A., Mumford, D. M. *et al.*: Epidemiologic findings and electron microscopic observations in human leukemia and canine contacts. *Int. J. Cancer*, **3**:7, 1968.

Vianna, N. J., Davies, J. N. P., Polan, A. *et al.*: Familial Hodgkin's disease: an environmental and genetic disorder. *Lancet*, **2**:854, 1974.

Vianna, N. J., Greenwald, P. and Davies, J. N. P.: Nature of the Hodgkin's disease agent. *Lancet*, **1**:733, 1971.

Vianna, N. J., Polan, A. K., Keogh, M. D. *et al.*: Hodgkin's disease mortality among physicians. *Lancet*, **2**:131, 1974.

Wald, N., Borges, W. H., Li, C. C. *et al.*: Leukemia associated with mongolism. *Lancet*, **1**:1228, 1961.

Waldman, T. A., Strober, W. and Blaese, R.: Immunodeficiency disease and malignancy. Various immunologic deficiencies of man and the role of immune processes in the control of malignant disease. *Ann. Int. Med.*, **77**:605, 1972.

Wells, R. and Law, K. S.: Incidence of leukemia in Singapore, and rarity of chronic lymphocytic leukemia in Chinese. *Brit. Med. J.*, **1**:759, 1960.

Index